Praise for
Pandemics and Peace:
Public Health Cooperation in Zones of Conflict

"This book is an original and unique contribution to the literature on infectious disease detection and response, offering an encyclopedic consideration of regional health diplomacy as a 'bridge to peace.' The volume presents a very detailed case study of three transnational regional disease surveillance programs of varying effectiveness and tackles the question of the legitimacy and accountability of the transnational public-private partnerships which play an increasingly central role in global health assistance."
—**Julie Fischer,** Stimson Center

"Disease threatens economic and social stability, increasing despair and the potential for violence in any country. Yet, I've seen firsthand how strong national and international partnerships and community-driven health efforts, like the Guinea worm eradication campaign, can be unexpected vehicles for peace in areas of long-standing conflict. Pandemics and Peace *outlines what's possible when we work together for the common good and is a valuable resource for scholars and field implementers."*
—**John B. Hardman, MD,** president and CEO, The Carter Center

"It is surprising that no one had written this needed book before. But now we have it, and Pandemics and Peace *greatly enriches our understanding of how, when, and why medical cooperation occurs even in the face of international conflict."*
—**Robert Jervis,** Adlai E. Stevenson Professor of International Politics, Columbia University

"This excellent book is rich in information and insight, comprehensively conceived, with wise and timely policy suggestions. Long provides a detailed analysis of three regional organizations that cooperatively conduct infectious disease surveillance programs that function among countries with contentious relations in the Middle East, Southeast Asia, and East Africa. This is an admirable work based on solid research and a thorough use of relevant theories."
—**Louis Kriesberg,** Maxwell Professor Emeritus of Social Conflict Studies, Syracuse University

"This volume provides a very good overview of trends in international health interdependencies and collaboration among a variety of actors to stem harmful impacts. Of particular note is the influence of health interdependencies on security interests and the evolution of the activities of varied actors. There are particularly interesting commentaries on the roles of nonstate actors. These actors include intergovernmental organizations and commercial and humanitarian bodies. The study is quite readable and should be purchased by a wide range of individuals and groups in the health and international relations fields."
—**Mark Zacher,** professor emeritus of political science and former director of the Institute of International Relations at University of British Columbia

PANDEMICS AND PEACE

PANDEMICS AND PEACE

PUBLIC HEALTH COOPERATION IN ZONES OF CONFLICT

WILLIAM J. LONG

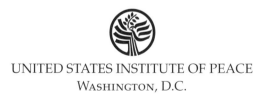

UNITED STATES INSTITUTE OF PEACE
WASHINGTON, D.C.

United States Institute of Peace
2301 Constitution Aveue, NW
Washington, DC 20037
www.usip.org

First published 2011

Printed in the United States of America

The paper used in this publication meets the minimum requirements of American National Standards for Information Science—Permanence of Paper for Printed Library Materials, ANSI Z39.48-1984.

Library of Congress Cataloging-in-Publication Data

Long, William J., 1956-
    Pandemics and peace : public health cooperation in zones of conflict / William J. Long.
        p. cm.
    Includes bibliographical references and index.
    ISBN 978-1-60127-080-1 (pbk. : alk. paper)
    1. Public health--Mekong River Delta (Vietnam and Cambodia)--International cooperation. 2. Public health--Middle East--International cooperation. 3. Public health--Africa, East--International cooperation. 4. Public health--International cooperation--Case studies. 5. War--Medical aspects. I. United States Institute of Peace. II. Title.
    RA441.L66 2011
    362.1--dc22
                                    2010046894

for Mary B.

CONTENTS

FOREWORD

Five years ago, bird flu broke out in the Middle East. Health professionals from Israel, Palestine, and Jordan contained its spread by
working together and sharing information. This cooperation continued even during outbreaks of regional violence in 2006 and 2009. When
swine flu was discovered in Israel in May 2009, just a few months after the
Gaza war, health officials from all three governments met and implemented
a plan they had developed over the past three years. Conflict in the Middle
East is not surprising; cooperation is, especially when it comes on the heels
of hot war and not just 'normal' tensions.

In so many respects William Long's *Pandemics and Peace: Public Health
Cooperation in Zones of Conflict* is an important book. The threat posed by
pandemics in a globalized world has only begun to be given its due. We've
had our scares so far: SARS, H1N1, avian flu. A combination of good
fortune—the H1N1 strand was not as severe as it could have been—and
effective policies have contained their impacts. But the 'DMD' potential—
diseases of mass destruction—remains ominous. The first chapter of the
book presents a valuable overarching discussion of this global public health
challenge, reviewing the literature in a comprehensive fashion as well as
providing the author's own insights.

As difficult as pandemic prevention is as an overall global policy challenge, it is that much more difficult in zones of conflict. Any author who
takes on the hard cases is to be commended. It makes demonstrating positive findings that much more difficult. But it makes any such findings all
the more significant. Long's book bears both points out. Along with the
Israel-Palestine-Jordan case, he includes such other conflict regions as the

Balkans, Mekong River Delta, East Africa, and Southern Africa. Each is an empirically rich case built on impressive field research as well as relevant official documents, other studies, and well-mined interdisciplinary literature, showing what the parties have been doing and how they've been doing it.

By working with tough test cases, Long also is able to engage core debates in the international relations literature over theories of cooperation. He captures the '-isms' debate as among interests (realism), institutions (liberalism), and identity (constructivism). He is diligent in presenting and testing his hypotheses against the data and the explanations that flow from the respective theories. In so doing he avoids the oft-played academic version of king-of-the-hill, of my theory is right and yours wrong, with a 'pieces of the puzzle' integration that is true to complexity without falling back into all theories having equal explanatory power. This approach makes the book quite useful for graduate international relations core courses, as well as for studying global public health.

The fact that the book combines this scholarly value with genuine policy relevance gives it added value in 'bridging the gap' efforts. The chapter on U.S. policy provides a comprehensive survey of relevant elements of U.S. global health policy with particular focus on those most influential for pandemic prevention. The analysis is balanced, giving credit where due and being critical as warranted. The policy recommendations are pitched at a level consistent with the nature of the book, not so general as to lack applicable guidance but also not professing to be the kind of full action plan that requires intragovernmental information and context. As such, the book manifests the mission to which the U.S. Institute of Peace is committed and contributes to efforts of others of us within the academy to enhance policy relevance.[1]

A lot of authors claim 'immense practical and theoretical significance'— Bill Long justifiably makes this claim. This is a rich and significant book.

—Bruce W. Jentleson
Duke University

---

1. Bruce W. Jentleson and Ely Ratner, "Bridging the Beltway-Ivory Tower Gap," *International Studies Review* 13, no. 2 (March 2011); Bruce W. Jentleson, "The Need for Praxis: Bringing Policy Relevance Back In," *International Security* 26, no. 4 (Spring 2002). See also the "Bridging the Gap" Project that I have initiated along with colleagues at Duke, UC Berkeley and the George Washington University Elliott School, http://www.gwu.edu/~btg/.

ACKNOWLEDGMENTS

This book benefited from the support and guidance of many individuals and institutions. In particular, I thank the Jennings Randolph Senior Scholars Program of the United States Institute of Peace under the leadership of Dr. Chantal de Jonge Oudraat, for its support. Backing for this work also came from my academic home, the Sam Nunn School of International Affairs at the Georgia Institute of Technology; the MacArthur Foundation; the East-West Center; and the United Nations Development Program.

The book would not have been possible without the insights of many, many individuals in the U.S. government, international organizations, nongovernmental organizations, and academic institutions who provided insights and direction to my study. I benefited also from the thorough reading and helpful comments of the three external reviewers of the manuscript. Any errors and omission in the text are purely my responsibility.

My thanks to Alexander Chapman, Meagan Clem, Jennifer Marsh, and Fred Plan for their careful and capable research assistance and to Wanda Moore for the preparation of the manuscript. Finally, my unending appreciation and love to my family for their encouragement and support.

ACRONYMS

AFENET	African Field Epidemiology Network
AFHSC	Armed Forces Health Surveillance Center
AFRO	World Health Organization Regional Office for Africa
AIDS	Acquired Immune Deficiency Syndrome
ASEAN	Association of Southeast Asian Nations
CDC	Centers for Disease Control and Prevention
CHORDS	Connecting Health Organizations for Regional Disease Surveillance
CMC	Cooperative Monitoring Center
CSIS	Center for Strategic and International Studies
DEISS	Division of Emerging Infectious and Surveillance Services (IDSR)
DESCD	Division of Epidemiology and Surveillance Capacity Development (IDSR)
DOD	U.S. Department of Defense
EAC	East African Community
EAIDSNet	East African Integrated Disease and Surveillance Network
EB	Executive Board
EPIET	European Program for Intervention Epidemiology Training
FAO	UN Food and Agricultural Organization
FDA	U.S. Food and Drug Administration
FELTP	Field Epidemiological and Laboratory Training Program

FETP	Field Epidemiology Training Program
GAO	U.S. Government Accountability Office
GDD	Global Disease Detection Program
GEIS	Global Emerging Infections Surveillance and Response System
GHI	Global Health Initiative
GHSI	Global Health and Security Initiative
GID	Global Immunization Division (IDSR)
GIS	Geographic Information Systems
GOARN	Global Outbreak and Response Network
GPHIN	Global Public Health Intelligence Network
HHS	U.S. Department of Health and Human Services
HIV	Human Immunodeficiency Virus
H1N1	Novel Influenza A, "swine flu"
H5N1	Human Influenza A, "bird flu"
ICT	Information and Communications Technologies
IDSR	Integrated Disease Surveillance and Response Program
IHE	Integrating the Healthcare Enterprise
IHR	International Health Regulations
INGO	international nongovernmental organization
LNHO	League of Nations Health Organization
MBDS	Mekong Basin Disease Surveillance Network
MBDSC	Mekong Basin Disease Surveillance Cooperation
MECIDS	Middle East Consortium on Infectious Disease Surveillance
MOU	Memorandum of Understanding
NGO	nongovernmental organization
NIMR	Tanzania National Institute for Medical Research

NSTC-7	National Science and Technology Council, Executive Office of the President, Presidential Decision Directive
NTI	Nuclear Threat Initiative
OIE	World Organization for Animal Health
PAHO	Pan American Health Organization
PEPFAR	President's Emergency Plan for AIDS Relief
PHEIC	Public Health Emergencies of International Concern
PHIAD	Public Health Information Affinity Domain
PPP	public-private partnership
ProMED	Program for Monitoring Emerging Diseases
SACIDS	South African Center for Infectious Disease Surveillance
SARS	Severe Acute Respiratory Syndrome
SEEHN	South-eastern Europe Health Network
SFCG	Search for Common Ground
SIT	Social Identity Theory
TEPHINET	Training Programs in Epidemiology and Public Health Interventions Network
TNC	transnational corporation
UNICEF	United Nations Children's Fund
UNSIC	United Nations System Influenza Coordination
USAID	U.S. Agency for International Development
USDA	U.S. Department of Agriculture
WHO	World Health Organization

1

PANDEMIC PEACE?

W hen bird flu broke out in the Middle East, Israeli, Palestinian, and Jordanian health officials worked side by side sharing information to prevent its spread. Networked cooperation among health professionals in the three locations in detecting, identifying, and monitoring infectious diseases made this successful response to a potential emergency possible.[1] Close collaboration continued even during the outbreaks of violence in the region in 2006 and 2009, so that when swine flu was reported in Israel in May 2009, health officials from the three jurisdictions met immediately at the Allenby Bridge, which links Jordan and Jerusalem, to implement a plan they had developed over the previous three years.[2] Likewise, the six countries of the Mekong River Basin—a region of numerous interstate wars in the recent past—have worked together quietly for more than a decade to coordinate surveillance and response to air- and waterborne diseases, including the deadly avian influenza.[3] Countries in conflict-prone or resource-poor regions such as East Africa,[4] Southern

---

1. Cooperation among the three entities occurs under the auspices of the Middle East Consortium on Infectious Disease Surveillance (MECIDS).
2. Louise Gresham et al., "Trust Across Borders: Responding to the H1N1 Influenza in the Middle East," *Biosecurity and Bioterrorism: Biodefense Strategy, Practice, and Science* 7, no. 4 (2009): 399–404; Dale Gavlak, "Catching Outbreaks Wherever They Occur," *World Health Organization Bulletin* 87, no. 10 (October 2009): 741–42, who.int/bulletin/volumes/87/10/09-031009/en/.
3. The six countries are Cambodia, China, Laos, Myanmar, Thailand, and Vietnam and the organization is known as the Mekong Basin Disease Surveillance network (MDBS).
4. The East African Integrated Disease Surveillance Network (EAIDSNet) is a collaborative effort of the Ministries of Health of Kenya, Tanzania, and Uganda established under the auspices of the East African Community in 2003. Rwanda and Burundi joined the Community in 2007 and the Health Sub-Sector in 2009.

Africa,[5] and the Balkans[6] also are beginning to cooperate on infectious disease surveillance and response.

Although largely unnoticed, this form of international cooperation has immense practical and theoretical significance. Theoretically, these sub-regional initiatives present intriguing anomalies to the classic problem of interstate cooperation in providing a global or transnational public good[7] (health) in "anarchy."[8] In parts of the world with difficult histories, where trust is low and misunderstanding and recrimination high among countries, cooperation in an area of national vulnerability is especially provocative. It raises the question of why public health cooperation is occurring there. To answer this question, this book uses three unlikely cases—the Mekong Basin, the Middle East, and East Africa—to explore empirically and comparatively several contending but untested hypotheses suggested by the global health diplomacy literature.[9] In so doing, it develops an empirically grounded theoretical explanation that illustrates exactly how interests, institutions, and ideas together enable international cooperation. This explanation helps clarify the potential and problems of fostering transnational cooperation in international affairs in this and potentially a host of other important areas, such as counterterrorism, environmental challenges, resource management, human rights protection, and economic assistance.

Some might argue that cooperation in health is a lesser form of international cooperation and hence less relevant to understanding cooperation in

---

5.   The Southern African Center for Infectious Disease (SACIDS) is an emerging network of national institutions and research organizations involved in infectious disease surveillance. SACIDS brings together human, animal, and plant health sector experts from five countries—Democratic Republic of Congo, Mozambique, Tanzania, Zambia, and South Africa. SACIDS began operations in January 2008.

6.   The signatories of the Dubrovnik Pledge of 2001 conceived the South-Eastern Europe Health Network (SEEHN). Members of SEEHN include Albania, Bosnia and Herzegovina, Bulgaria, Croatia, Romania, Serbia and Montenegro, and the former Yugoslav Republic of Macedonia. A year later, cooperation was extended to Moldova and three regional donors: Greece, Hungary, and Slovenia. The primary aims of SEEHN are to increase the integration of regional health services, strengthen disease surveillance and control, and establish networks for information collection and sharing.

7.   Global public goods are benefits that are both nonexcludable and nonrival, and, though immensely desirable, they are chronically underprovided. See Scott Barrett, *Why Cooperate? The Incentive to Supply Global Public Goods* (New York: Oxford University Press, 2007).

8.   For a discussion of this term in international relations theory, see Alexander Wendt, "Anarchy Is What States Make of It: The Social Construction of Power Politics," *International Organization* 46, no. 2 (Spring 1992): 391–425.

9.   See, for example, Ilona Kickbusch, Gaudenz Silberschmidt, and Paulo Buss, "Global Health Diplomacy: The Need for New Perspectives, Strategic Approaches and Skills in Global Health," *World Health Organization Bulletin* 85, no. 3 (March 1987): 161–244, www.who.int/bulletin/volumes/85/3/06-039222/en/; Martin McKee, Paul Garner, and Robin Scott, eds., *International Cooperation and Health* (Oxford: Oxford University Press, 2001); Graeme MacQueen and Joanna Santa-Barbara, "Peacebuilding Through Health Initiatives," *British Medical Journal* 321 (2000): 293–96.

the most critical areas of international relations. I disagree. For example, in discussing new forms of transnational politics, Edgar Grande and Louis Pauly use the term *meso-politics* to refer to welfare-related issues (such as health) that follow security and foreign policy in importance but precede technical standardization.[10] As I argue in the next section of this chapter and later in chapter 5, infectious disease threat is now a first-order problem affecting both the security and welfare of states and the international system.[11]

Such is the conclusion of the World Health Organization (WHO), the U.S. government, and most scholars and policy practitioners. Moved by the severity of the threat to human and national security, in 2005 the 193 members states of the World Health Assembly (WHA) concluded a decade-long effort to overhaul its requirements for disease surveillance reporting and response, and set a strict timetable for implementation by its members. These requirements, discussed in chapter 2, greatly expanded both the number of diseases and threats that must be monitored and the responsibility of every state to meet these threats through national policies and participation in regional and global efforts. These changes are the first significant revision of the international health regulations in fifty years and the first expansion of the disease coverage since international agreements began in 1851. This comprehensive response to the spread of infectious disease, compared with the failed one to global warming, for example, attests to the consensus that states see this issue as a fundamental threat to their interests and are willing to devote substantial diplomatic and material resources to fighting it and to urging other states and regional organizations to fight it too.

Combating infectious disease has also become a top security concern of national policymakers and analysts. The 2000 U.S. National Intelligence Estimate, for example, classified infectious disease for the first time as a threat to national security: "new and reemerging infectious diseases will pose a rising global health threat and will complicate US and global security."[12] The

---

10. Edgar Grande and Louis W. Pauly, "Complex Sovereignty and the Emergence of Transnational Authority," in *Complex Sovereignty: Reconstituting Political Authority in the Twenty-First Century*, eds. Edgar Grande and Louis W. Pauly (Toronto: University of Toronto Press, 2005), 292–93. Regional cooperation in infectious disease control is a mid-level problem in the sense of falling between bilateral and fully multilateral cooperation and in the sense that the actors involved, though state agents, often do not attract the same level of public scrutiny as officials whose sole function is to represent state interests in matters of traditional security and foreign affairs.

11. See Harley Feldbaum et al., "Global Health and National Security: The Need for Critical Engagement" (unpublished manuscript, Center on Global Change and Health, London School of Hygiene and Tropical Medicine, 2004).

12. National Intelligence Council, "The Global Infectious Disease Threat and its Implications for the United States," NIE 99-17D (Washington, DC: National Intelligence Council, 2000), www.dni.gov/nic/special_globalinfectious.html.

2010 National Security Strategy reaffirms this concern.[13] Leading military and security policy experts have reached the same conclusions,[14] and in his recent book Andrew Price-Smith captures the academic consensus that epidemic disease "presents a direct threat to the power of the state, as it erodes prosperity, destabilizing the relations between state and society, renders institutions sclerotic, foments intrastate violence, and ultimately diminishes the power and cohesion of the state."[15]

Because the key participants in each of these transnational networks include public actors (states and international organizations) and private actors (nongovernmental organizations, transnational corporations, and philanthropies), this study also offers an opportunity to examine crucial questions in the field of public-private transnational governance.[16] Specifically, this book responds to two fundamental questions in the nascent literature: Are these new forms of governance effective in delivering transnational public goods and what factors contribute to or impede their effectiveness? Do these hybrid (public-private) international actors exercise political authority legitimately—that is, are they democratically accountable—and what factors enhance or detract from their legitimacy? The answers to these questions will generate working hypotheses on transnational networked governance for further investigation by scholars of global governance, and offer a plausible framework for practitioners and policymakers engaged in safeguarding this particular dimension of national and international security and welfare. Furthermore, these cases afford an occasion to examine the origins of transnational networks and to consider how they relate to states and international governmental organizations operating in the same policy arenas.

---

13. The White House, *National Security Strategy of the United States of America, May 2010* (Washington, DC: Executive Office of the President, 2010), 48–49, www.whitehouse.gov/sites/default/files/rss_viewr/national_security_strategy.pdf.

14. See, for example, Susan Peterson, "Epidemic Disease and National Security," *Security Studies* 12, no. 2 (2002): 43–81; Jennifer Brower and Peter Chalk, *The Global Threat of New and Reemerging Infectious Diseases: Reconciling U.S. National Security and Public Health Policy* (Santa Monica, CA: RAND Corporation, 2003); Michael Moodie and William J. Taylor Jr., "Contagion and Conflict: Health as a Global Security Challenge," Report of the Chemical and Biological Arms Control Institute and the Center for Strategic and International Studies, International Security Programs (Washington, DC: Center for Strategic and International Studies, 2000).

15. Andrew T. Price-Smith, *Contagion and Chaos: Disease Ecology and National Security in the Era of Globalization* (Cambridge, MA: MIT Press, 2009), 2.

16. Transnationalism refers to "regular interactions across national boundaries when at least one actor is a non-state agent." Networks are "forms of organization characterized by voluntary, reciprocal, and horizontal patterns of communication." See Robert Keohane and Joseph Nye, Jr., "Transnational Relations and World Politics: An Introduction," in *Transnational Relations and World Politics*, eds. Robert Keohane and Joseph Nye Jr., xi–xvi (Cambridge, MA: Harvard University Press, 1971).

Challenges and Opportunities Posed by Infectious Disease

The spread of avian influenza and other naturally occurring or man-made biological threats presents a grave security and humanitarian threat regionally and globally.[17] Dramatic increases in the worldwide movement of people, animals, and goods; growing population density; and uneven public health systems worldwide are the driving forces behind heightened vulnerability to the spread of both old and new infectious diseases.[18] Since the global spread of the human immunodeficiency virus (HIV) began in the early 1980s, twenty-nine new bacteria or viruses have been identified, many of which are capable of global reach.[19] Commenting on this trend in 2007, the United Nations' World Health Organization warned, "Since the 1970s, newly emerging diseases have been identified at the unprecedented rate of one or more per year. . . . It would be extremely naïve and complacent to assume that there will not be another disease like AIDS, another Ebola, or another SARS, sooner or later."[20] Senior World Health officials have noted that "inadequate surveillance and response capacity in a single country can endanger national populations and public health security of the entire world."[21]

With more than a million travelers flying across national boundaries every day, it is not an exaggeration to say that a health problem in any part of the world can rapidly become a health threat to many or all[22]—what one author calls the microbial unification of the world.[23] The outbreak of severe acute respiratory syndrome (SARS) in 2002 and 2003 demonstrated how a previously unknown but lethal virus could spread by modern air transport, traveling from Hong Kong to Toronto in fifteen hours and eventually

---

17. For an early discussion of this emerging threat, see Laurie Garrett, *The Coming Plague: Newly Emerging Diseases in a World out of Balance* (New York: Penguin, 1995). For a skeptical view, see the comments of Dr. Peter Palese in "Science," panel session at CFR Symposium on Pandemic Influenza: Science, Economics, and Foreign Policy, Council on Foreign Relations, New York, October 16, 2009, www.cfr.org/project/1442/cfr_symposium_on_pandemic_influenza.html.

18. "Neither globalization nor the potential [health] threat posed by globalization is new," citing the European discovery of the Americas that led to a devastating loss of life among indigenous people. See Sarah Payne, "Globalization, Governance, and Health," in *Governance, Globalization and Public Policy*, eds. Patricia Kennett (Cheltenham, UK: Edward Elgar, 2008), 153. By some estimates, 90 percent of those deaths were attributed to contagious diseases for which native populations had no immunity.

19. Lincoln Chen, Tim Evans, and Richard Cash, "Health as a Global Public Good," in *Global Public Goods: International Cooperation in the 21st Century*, eds. Inge Kaul, Isabelle Grunberg, and Mark A. Sterns (New York: Oxford University Press, 1999), 288.

20. WHO, *World Health Report* 2007 (Geneva: World Health Organization, 2007).

21. David Heymann and Guenael Rodier, "Global Surveillance, National Surveillance, and SARS," *Emerging Infectious Diseases* 10, no. 2 (2004), www.medscape.com/viewarticle/467371.

22. Kelley Lee, *Globalization and Health* (New York: Palgrave, 2003); Maureen T. Upton, "Global Public Health Trumps the Nation-State," *World Policy Journal* (Fall 2004): 73–78.

23. Giovanni Berlinguer, "Health and Equity as a Primary Global Goal," *Development* 42, no. 2 (1999): 12–16.

reaching twenty-seven countries.[24] The increased speed of transmission also means that contagion is likely to be well established before governments and international organizations are aware of the presence of the disease.[25]

SARS, in turn, focused attention on the ability of public health systems worldwide to cope with an anticipated pandemic associated with the next major antigenic shift in the influenza A virus. Although the influenza A virus mutates regularly (antigenic drift), every decade or so the virus undergoes a major change, or shift, for which most people have little or no protection. The threat is magnified today by the ability of such diseases to spread worldwide very rapidly.[26] For example, since emerging in 1997, avian influenza—which to date has infected more than 400 people and killed more than 200—could create, if it becomes capable of human-to-human transmission as a new influenza A virus, a global pandemic of unprecedented lethality. Avian influenza could, if it becomes capable of human-to-human transmission as SARS did in 2002, kill somewhere between 200,000 to 16 million Americans. Countries with less robust public health systems would lose an even larger percentage of their population to such a disease.[27] The relatively benign H1N1, or swine flu, outbreak provides a harbinger of this future danger.

Global economic and political stability could fall victim to a pandemic too. Today, nations must provide for their citizens' health and well-being and protect them from disease. Health provision has become a primary public good and part of the social contract between a people and its government.[28] Accelerating transnational flows, especially pathogens, can stress and could overwhelm a state's capacity to meet this essential function. Weak states could fail economically or politically, thereby creating regional instability and a breeding ground for terrorism or human rights violations.[29] Statistical studies reveal that declining public health substantially increases the probability

---

24. Kelley Lee and Derek Yach, "Globalization and Health," in *International Public Health: Disease, Programs, Systems and Policies*, eds. Michael H. Merson, Robert E. Black, and Anne J. Mills (Sudbury, MA: Jones and Bartlett Publishers, 2006), 690.

25. Payne, "Globalization, Governance, and Health," 164.

26. Lee and Yach, "Globalization and Health," 689.

27. Global Alert and Response, "Pandemic Preparedness," World Health Organization, www.who.int/csr/disease/influenza/pandemic/en.

28. See Andrew Price-Smith, *The Health of Nations: Infectious Diseases, Environmental Change, and Their Effects on National Security* (Cambridge, MA: MIT Press, 2002). This state responsibility is not new. Historically, one of the first functions of the emerging trading states in the late Middle Ages was the development of maritime quarantine systems to protect their populations from importing diseases. See Kelley Lee, Susan Fustukian, and Kent Buse, "An Introduction to Global Health Policy," in *Health Policy in a Globalising World*, eds. Kelley Lee, Susan Fustukian, and Kent Buse (Cambridge: Cambridge University Press, 2002) 3–17.

29. Commission on Macroeconomics and Health, *Investing in Health* (Geneva: World Health Organization, 2003).

of state failure,[30] and historical examples of the correlation between disease outbreak and political instability and violence extend from the fall of ancient Athens to recent violence in Zimbabwe. Even in the strongest states, leaders must be prepared, in an integrated way, to respond to the full spectrum of biological threats that could impede essential social functions such as food supply, transportation, education, and workforce operation and result in huge economic costs.[31]

Reducing the danger of influenza or other infectious diseases requires a focus on preparedness and monitoring. Rapidly identifying the problem, sharing information, and coordinating response are each critical to limiting the perils of pathogenic threats. Although the peril is great, so too is the promise of building cooperation through regional disease surveillance, detection, and response.

Here is the positive potential of globalization: it can facilitate the rapid response to health challenges by quickly mobilizing health professionals, medicines, and supplies, and by deploying information technology for disease surveillance and sharing best health practices across nations.[32] These exchanges, between neighboring states and even between traditional adversaries, could contribute to reducing disparities in health and help improve regional relations. Armed with a theoretical understanding of the basis for such cooperation, the regional and international practitioner and policy communities can respond more effectively to this critical transnational security and humanitarian concern.[33]

---

30. See Gary King and Langche Zang, "Improving Forecasts of State Failure," *World Politics* 53, no. 4 (July 2001): 623–58, doi:10.1353/wp.2001.0018.

31. K. C. Decker and Keith Holtermann, "The Role for Exercises in Senior Policy Pandemic Influenza Preparedness," *Journal of Homeland Security and Emergency Management* 6, no. 1 (2009): 1–15, doi:10.2202/1547-7355.1521. The cost of an influenza pandemic in the United States has been estimated to be somewhere between $71.3 to $166.5 billion. Martin I. Meltzer, Nancy J. Cox, and Keiji Fukuda, "The Economic Impact of Pandemic Influenza in the United States: Priorities for Intervention," *Emerging Infectious Diseases* 5, no. 5 (1999): 659–71.

32. See Kelley Lee, "Globalization: A New Agenda for Health," in *International Cooperation in Health*, eds. Martin McKee, Paul Garner, and Robin Stott (Oxford: Oxford University Press, 2001), 13–30; Mark W. Zacher, "The Transformation in Global Health Collaboration since the 1990s," in *Governing Global Health: Challenge, Response, Innovation*, eds. Andrew Fenton Cooper, John J. Kirton, and Ted Schrecker (Burlington, VT: Ashgate Publishing, 2007) 15–27.

33. According the UNDP's human-centric definition, security involves protection from a range of threats including "disease, hunger, unemployment, crime, social conflict, political repression, and environmental hazards." See United Nations Development Program, *Human Development Report 1994* (New York: Oxford University Press, 1995), 22. This broader notion of security has become increasingly meaningful in practice, including state practice. See Armed Forces Health Surveillance Center, "Global Emerging Infectious Surveillance and Response Systems," (Washington, DC: U.S. Department of Defense), www.afhsc.nil/geisPartners. Many states, including the United States, consider the defense against infectious disease to be a part of their national security policy. See Feldbaum et al., "Global Health and National Security."

This chapter outlines general theories of interstate cooperation and how, to date, health practitioners, policymakers, and analysts have attempted to account for international cooperation in the global public health domain more particularly. These hypotheses provide pathways into the empirical investigation in chapter 2. Chapter 3 returns to the question of cooperation and develops a unique theoretical explanation for this anomaly that blends elements of our general understandings of the prospects and problems of international cooperation into an integrated and more specified theory of cooperation in health and potentially other arenas of international affairs.

Attempts to Explain International Cooperation in Public Health

Because states remain indispensable actors in these cases, international relations theory is a useful framework for thinking about international and transnational cooperation in public health and disease surveillance and response.[34] This literature is vast. In a nutshell, though political realism in its many forms emphasizes the enduring propensity for conflict among self-interested states seeking their security in an anarchic environment, that is, one where there is no central authority to protect states from each other or to guarantee their security. Hence international cooperation is thought to be rare, fleeting, and tenuous—limited by enforcement problems and each state's preferences for relative gains in their relationships because of their systemic vulnerability.[35] Liberal approaches are particularly interested in identifying several ways to mitigate the conflictive tendencies of international relations, particularly through shared economic interests and norms and institutions (e.g., democracy). Liberals argue that these factors can help ameliorate the enforcement problem in anarchy and permit states to focus more on mutual gain defined in absolute rather than relative terms.[36] More recently, constructivist approaches emphasize that nonmaterial, ideational factors, not just state interests and national and international institutions, are critical to understanding the formation of interests and the possibility

---

34. Transnationalism, as distinct from internationalism, implies that though states remain important or even indispensable actors, they find themselves drawn increasingly into nonhierarchical modes of governance involving both public and private actors. See Grande and Pauly, "Complex Sovereignty," 3–21.

35. Contemporary classics of political realism in its traditional and structural variants include Hans J. Morgenthau, *Politics among Nations: The Struggle for Power and Peace*, 3rd ed. (New York: Alfred A. Knopf, 1960); Kenneth N. Waltz, *Theory of International Politics* (Reading, MA: Addison-Wesley, 1979).

36. See, for example, Robert Keohane and Joseph Nye Jr., *Power and Interdependence*, 3rd ed. (New York: Longman, 2000).

of cooperation. As the name implies, for constructivists, the interests and identities of states are highly malleable and context-specific and the anarchic structure of the international system does not, in itself, dictate that conflict is the norm and cooperation the exception. Rather, the process of interaction between and among actors shapes how political actors (not just states) define themselves and their interests: "self-help and power politics do not follow logically or causally from anarchy. . . . Anarchy is what states make of it."[37] Because identities and interests are not dictated by structure, a state's purely egoistic interests can be transformed under anarchy to create collective identities and interests by intentional efforts and positive interaction.

Moving away from concerns about whether theory should focus primarily on interests, institutions, or ideas as the key causal variable in understanding cooperation (or the lack thereof), the theory of cooperation that emerges in chapter 3 blends elements of these and other approaches, often cast as alternatives, to demonstrate precisely the processes by which interests, institutions, and ideas (particularly about identity) can combine to shape cooperation in this, and arguably other, areas of international relations. In so doing, it demonstrates the organic interrelationship among the causal forces of cooperation and specifies the characteristics and dimensions of interests, institutions, and ideas about identity that facilitate cooperation.[38]

Most explanations for international cooperation in the area of public health come from practitioners, policymakers, and analysts, not international relations scholars.[39] To account for cooperation in matters of international public health, the practitioner and analyst literature offers several contending, but largely untested, proto-hypotheses that draw from various social science approaches:

- An interest-based argument derived from the forces of globalization and the social nature of the problem, that the global benefits from controlling the transnational spread of disease necessitate cooperation and that "enlightened self-interest and altruism will converge in the increasingly interdependent world being shaped by the process

---

37. Wendt, "Anarchy Is What States Make of It," 394–95.

38. On the value of blended explanations for understanding complex international dynamics see Richard Deeg and Mary O'Sullivan, "The Political Economy of Global Financial Capital," *World Politics* 61, no. 4 (October 2009): 731–63, doi:10.2202/1547-7355.1521.

39. Recently, scholars of international relations have begun to focus on issues in global health, some applying an explicitly theoretical perspective. See, for example, Mark W. Zacher and Tania J. Keefe, *The Politics of Global Health Governance: United by Contagion* (New York: Palgrave MacMillan, 2008); Price-Smith, *Contagion and Chaos*.

of globalization."[40] Infectious diseases know no physical borders and present particularly compelling superordinate problems that transcend the interests of contending parties, are shared by all of them, and require joint efforts for effective response.[41] This explanation identifies the potential basis for interest-based cooperation in infectious disease surveillance and response, but fails to address how the difficulties inherent in providing an international public good such as disease control are overcome.

- A psychosocial, identity hypothesis that health initiatives promote an environment that emphasizes human well-being. The aim of reducing pain and disease is relatively undisputed. Health initiatives thus help overcome other, more divisive sources of identity by shifting the focus away from questions of national or ethnic security to human security, and allowing for an evocation and extension of altruism.[42] How such identities are formed and reformed is not addressed, however.

- A scientism or epistemic community hypothesis that health cooperation creates a realm of objectivity and much-needed expertise in areas where propaganda, suspicion, and recrimination often dominate relations.[43] Medical experts can phrase the causes and the responses to health threats in scientific terms. Health workers, in turn, have greater credibility as unbiased professionals, thereby encouraging greater trust and reliance among actors from different states. For example, Martin McKee, Paul Garner, and Robin Stott assert that "health professionals thus have a unique combination of competence in communication, trust of civil society, intimate contact with most of the members thereof, and the capacity to influence individuals whatever their role in society."[44] These observations draw our attention to the critical issue of trust and how to establish and maintain it across borders.

40. Derek Yach and Douglas Bettcher, "The Globalization of Public Health, I: Threats and Opportunities," *American Journal of Public Health* 88, no. 5 (1998): 735–44.

41. See Ronald J. Fisher, *The Social Psychology of Intergroup and International Conflict Resolution* (New York: Springer-Verlag, 1990).

42. See Harvey Skinner et al., "Promoting Arab and Israeli Cooperation: Peacebuilding through Health Initiatives," *The Lancet* 365 (April 2, 2005): 1247–77.

43. Scientism suggests that certain socially beneficial, technical tasks should be handed over to experts. See Craig Murphy, "Global Governance: Poorly Done and Poorly Understood," in *The Global Governance Reader*, ed. Rorden Wilkinson, 90–104 (New York: Routledge, 2005). Epistemic community is a network among professionals with an authoritative claim to policy-relevant knowledge. See Peter M. Hass, "Knowledge, Power and International Policy Coordination," *International Organization* 46, no. 1 (1992): 1–35.

44. See Martin McKee, Paul Gardner, and Robin Scott, "Introduction," in *International Cooperation in Health* (Oxford: Oxford University Press, 2001), 10.

- A domestic politics, rational choice[45] hypothesis that health cooperation provides an essential national public good[46] (physical security) that
  redounds to a participating government's credit, thus enhancing state
  capacity and legitimacy and improving regional stability. This approach
  highlights the domestic, state-level, variables that might help account
  for cooperation. Furthermore, positive results in health can be observed
  and measured by epidemiological statistics on mortality and morbidity,
  have powerful impacts on citizens, and thus are attractive investments
  for governmental and nongovernmental actors.[47]
- A negotiation and signaling hypothesis that health initiatives, as voluntary, novel, and consequential projects, are reliable signals for improving communication, reducing threats, and breaking patterns of
  conflict among traditional rivals or antagonists.[48] For example, Thomas
  Novotny and Vincanne Adams maintain that "health and scientific interactions can serve as core diplomatic gestures to improve communication, reduce mutual or bilateral threats, and address health problems
  of mutual importance."[49] This observation suggests that health initiatives can be a top-down strategy as part of national statecraft.

Furthermore, drawing from functionalist and neofunctionalist theory, the
public health diplomacy literature suggests that health sector cooperation
can spillover into other technical areas (natural disaster planning, for example) or even sensitive political and security arenas (mitigating man-made
biological threats, for instance).[50] Is this so, and what would explain health as
the leading edge of wider cooperation?

---

45. Assumptions of rational decision making are as follows: actors pursue goals; these goals reflect
the actor's perceived interests; behavior results from a process that involves, or functions as if it entails,
conscious choice; the individual is the basic agent in society; actors have preferences that are consistent
and stable; if given options, actors will choose the alternative with the highest expected utility; and
actors possess extensive information on both the available alternatives and the likely consequences of
their choices. These assumptions apply with equal force for all persons.

46. Unlike international public goods, national public goods are more likely to be provided through the
use of governmental coercion. See Barrett, *Why Cooperate?* This issue is addressed in detail in chapter 3.

47. Judith Richter, "Public-Private Partnerships for Health: A Trend with No Alternatives?" *Development* 47, no. 2 (2004): 43–48.

48. See James D. Fearon, "Domestic Political Audiences and the Escalation of International Disputes," *American Political Science Review* 88 (1994): 577–92.

49. Vincanne Adams and Thomas Novotny, "Global Health Diplomacy" (working paper, Global
Health Sciences, University of California, San Francisco, January 16, 2007), 1–10.

50. According to David Mitrany, technological issues confronting modern industrialized nations in
the twentieth century require international cooperation along functional lines. He suggests that organizations for functional cooperation will eventually eclipse the political institutions of the past such as
the national state. See David Mitrany, *A Working Peace System. An Argument for the Functional Development of International Organization* (Chicago: University of Chicago Press, 1943, 1966). Arguing from a
neofunctionalist perspective, Ernst Hass maintained that rational behavior led not only to transnational

Using evidence from the cases of the Mekong Basin Disease Surveillance Network (MBDS), the Middle East Consortium on Infectious Disease Surveillance (MECIDS), and the East Africa Integrated Disease Surveillance Network (EAIDSNet), this book investigates whether there is support for any of these notions or some elements of them, and determines how these instances of cooperation fit within and speak to our understanding of broad theories of international cooperation.

Transnational Governance: Examining Public-Private Partnerships

Governments acting alone cannot meet the challenge of infectious disease spread. Diseases cross and even ignore the geopolitical boundaries of the state. The six countries of the Mekong Basin share thousands of miles of borderlands and waterways crossed by more than a million people a year. Eighty miles separate the capitals of Jordan, Israel, and the Palestine Authority, and the five nations of the East African Integrated Disease Surveillance Network are similarly intertwined. Effective disease surveillance and response must also cross borders and requires not just governments, but governance.[51] *Governance* can be defined as the "ability to promote collective action and deliver collective decisions"[52] and, as distinct from government, can be fulfilled by a wide range of individuals and institutions including the public sector, private companies, nongovernmental organizations, professional bodies, and civil society.[53] An investigation into regional or global governance cannot slight the interests of traditional national actors or the distribution of power in a given policy arena, but must also consider other actors that might facilitate cooperation and the role that knowledge and norms play in managing a particular problem.

In health, power has shifted from vertically organized governments and international agencies to horizontally linked coalitions or networks that also include private actors such as nongovernmental organizations, businesses, and philanthropies; a process of institutional pluralism driven by changing ideological and institutional preferences, technological advances, new sources

---

interdependence, but also to the creation of supranational institutions, such as the European Community, which contribute to international peace. See *The Uniting of Europe: Political, Social, and Economic Sources 1950–1957* (Stanford, CA: Stanford University Press, 1958).

51. McKee, Gardner, and Scott, "Introduction," 21.

52. Richard Dodgson, Kelley Lee, and Nick Drager, "Global Health Governance: A Conceptual Review," in *Global Health Governance: Key Issues*, ed. Kelley Lee (Westport, CT: Greenwood Press, 2000), 6.

53. McKee, Gardner, and Scott, "Introduction."

of funding; and lower barriers to entry.[54] These new amalgamations have been labeled global health alliances, global health partnerships, and global public-private partnerships.[55] The three examples of public-private governance initiatives in infectious disease control examined in this study provide a basis for systematically exploring key questions regarding global health governance, and transnational problem-solving networks.[56] Specifically, we want to know whether these experiments in transnational governance can collectively solve problems and effectively deliver the (public) goods. If so, we need to identify the factors that either are necessary or facilitate effective governance. In addition, we want to use these cases both to consider whether the authority wielded by these transnational networks is legitimate, defined in terms of democratic accountability, and specify the factors that enhance or impede their legitimacy.

Detailed comparative analysis of the governance process in these three cases will generate useful insights for practitioners and researchable hypotheses for scholars. For practitioners and policymakers, generic insights can be tailored to their specific circumstances. For scholars and students, these cases may contribute to a better understanding of global governance, private-public partnerships, and transnational problem-solving networks by generating plausible hypotheses about the effectiveness, legitimacy, and origins of transnational networks for further inquiry.

---

54.   Rene Loewenson, "Civil Society Influence on Global Health Policy" (online report, Geneva: World Health Organization, 2003), www.tarsc.org/WHOCSI/globalhealth.php. See also Marco Schäferhoff, Sabine Campe, and Christopher Kaan, "Transnational Public-Private Partnerships in International Relations: Making Sense of Concepts, Research Frameworks, and Results," *International Studies Review* 11 (2009): 451–74; Nirmala Ravishankar et al., "Financing Global Health: Tracking Development Assistance for Health from 1990 to 2007," *The Lancet* 373 (June 20, 2009): 2113–24.

55.   See also Zacher and Keefe, *Politics of Global Health Governance*, 7; Kent Buse and Gill Walt, "Global Public-Private Partnerships: Part II, What Are the Health Issues for Global Governance," *Bulletin of the World Health Organization* 78, no. 5 (2005), www.who.int/bulletin/archives/78(5)699.pdf.

56.   Global health governance is defined as collective action to deliver cooperative solutions in the pursuit of common goals in health. See Richard Dodgson, Kelley Lee, and Nick Drager, "Global Health Governance: A Conceptual Review" (Geneva: World Health Organization and London School of Hygiene and Tropical Medicine, 2002); David P. Fidler, "Architecture amidst Anarchy: Global Health's Quest for Governance," *Global Health Governance* 1, no. 1 (January 2007). Transnational problem-solving networks are defined as relevant actors working internationally on an issue, bound together by shared values, a common discourse, and dense exchanges of information. See Margaret Keck and Kathryn Sikkink, *Activists beyond Borders: Advocacy Networks in International Politics* (Ithaca, NY: Cornell University Press, 1998). Jean-François Rischard has argued that networked governance has two generic features that rectify limitations of the current international system: they have a minimum of bureaucracy with a maximum of knowledge; and relatedly, their start up and delivery time are fast-aiming for global action, not global legislation. See Jean-François Rischard, "Global Issue Networks: Desperate Times Deserve Innovative Measures," *The Washington Quarterly* 26, no. 1 (2003): 17–33.

Thoughts on Policy and Practice

As noted, the fight against infectious disease spread occurs on many levels: global, pan-regional, subregional, and national and these initiatives are inter-dependent. Chapter 2 introduces the global and pan-regional frameworks for fighting infectious disease and analyzes in-depth the working of three intriguing subregional infectious disease control networks. National policies are also critical in infectious disease control and, as discussed at length in chapter 5, no nation is more important than the United States in this respect. The United States, as a leader in both medical and information technology, is well situated to strengthen public health systems abroad and indirectly support regional health cooperation as a peaceful and positive dimension of its global health diplomacy and a frontline defense of its own population from the threat of infectious diseases, outbreaks of which typically begin in the developing world. Beyond terrorism, disease surveillance and response provides the United States an opportunity to address a critical national and transnational problem. Indeed, because it is largely apolitical and nonreligious, combating pandemics, more than counterterrorism, may offer a basis on which to build better bilateral relations and lay a foundation for regional cooperation. The U.S. government could, by helping prevent the political and social discord and the personal suffering wrought by pandemic disease, win the good will of both foreign governments and peoples.

To date, some domestic actors—notably the U.S. Centers for Disease Control and Prevention (CDC), the U.S. Department of Defense (DOD), and the United States Agency for International Development (USAID)—have participated indirectly in support of some of these subregional networks by their assistance to infectious disease surveillance and response capacity abroad. Chapter 5 analyses in detail the programs of the U.S. government explicitly designed to bolster foreign capacity in infectious disease control within the larger context of America's global health diplomacy. It asks whether the policies and the institutional arrangements of the U.S. government are enough to fully meet the challenge that infectious disease spread poses to national and international security and whether the United States is doing all it should to maximize the potential diplomatic benefits to be had from its policies.

Method and Design

This study, using a detailed, theoretically informed, comparative case design, considers why cooperation is occurring and what factors facilitate or impede the success of transnational organizations. An in-depth study of a few cases provides an opportunity to explore these questions contextually yet systematically. Although less parsimonious than some approaches, case method can lead to plausible statements of causality regarding why and how health-based cooperation is occurring in complicated regions when many variables are involved.[57] A situated approach yields an added advantage: insights that may prove helpful to policymakers and practitioners accustomed to wrestling with real world complexities and ambiguities.[58]

This methodology presents certain challenges, of course. The most significant is the problem of complex, multiple determinants of social phenomena and the risk of spurious or invalid inferences being drawn from a few cases in which many causal factors may be at play—in short, overdeterminacy.[59] To control for this, the investigation is defined by systematic use of the hypotheses about the possible reasons for health policy cooperation and the central debates on transnational public-private governance and a within-case process-tracing procedure.

In terms of data collection, multiple sources of evidence are used to strengthen construct validity. Data sources include semistructured interviews, field and participant observations, and document and archival analysis.

Regarding case selection, each of the disease surveillance networks studied is an important policy initiative, and two of the three are dramatic examples of subregional cooperation. In general, the cases are what we call least-likely instances, given the absence of favorable factors such as existing institutions, regimes, or normative consensus, and because infectious disease control requires that states share sensitive information about the vulnerability of their populations and the weaknesses of their institutions. These cases may thus tell us something unique and important about the possibilities and mechanisms for international cooperation generally. For controlled comparison and to reduce selection bias, some significant variance exits along the dependent variables (cooperation and governance effectiveness and legitimacy): MBDS as the most established institutionally, MECIDS as less codified but highly effective, and EAIDSNet as much less successful in sustaining cooperation in infectious disease monitoring and response. The fieldwork for the cases was

57. Gary King, Robert Keohane, and Sidney Verba, *Designing Social Inquiry* (Princeton, NJ: Princeton University Press, 1994).

58. Alexander L. George, *Bridging the Gap: Theory and Practice in Foreign Policy* (Washington, DC: U.S. Institute of Peace, 2003); Alexander George and Andrew Bennett, *Case Studies and Theory Development in the Social Sciences* (Cambridge, MA: Massachusetts Institute of Technology, 2005).

59. Robert K. Yin, *Case Study Research: Design and Methods* (Beverly Hills, CA: Sage Publications, 1989).

conducted sequentially with the first—MBDS—establishing the theoretical boundaries of the study and related interview and other data protocols.

Organization of the Book

Chapter 2 provides a brief consideration of the global governance framework for infectious disease surveillance and response, a detailed discussion of the three case studies, and a look at a very recent effort to link these three regional networks and other similar networks together in an organization known as CHORDS (Connecting Health Organizations for Regional Disease Surveillance).

Chapter 3 draws from the empirical investigation to distill a unique theoretical explanation for the processes by which interests, institutions, and ideas can align to enable international cooperation even in difficult circumstances. This approach, I suggest, may have potentially broader relevance for appreciating, explaining, and encouraging other critically important but less visible forms of regional interstate cooperation, and it moves us away from what one scholar calls "the Olympian interpretation of relations among states,"[60] toward more meaningful understanding of real-world cooperation in a regional context.

Chapter 4 focuses on transnational problem-solving networks, in particular public-private partnerships. Here the emphasis is to generate working hypotheses about this new and important phenomenon in world politics. A growing list of polemical works on transnational networks casts them as everything from the answer to global problems to the scourge of democratic principles and the perpetuation of corporate control over the world's poor.[61] Most of these works are based on anecdotal evidence or single case studies collected in edited volumes. This study both sheds light on issues related to the effectiveness, legitimacy, and operation of transnational problem-solving networks and public-private partnerships and hones propositions about their operation and effects that scholars can use for further investigation and practitioners can refine for particular policy purposes. Developing workable hypotheses about the origins, operation, and factors that enhance or impede the success of transnational public-private networks is the goal of chapter 4.

---

60. I. William Zartman, "Dialog of the Deaf, Mutual Enlightenment or Doing One's Own Thing?" paper presented at the Annual Conference of the International Studies Association, New Orleans, LA (February 18, 2010).

61. Compare Wolfgang H. Reinicke and Francis Deng, *Critical Choices: United Nations, Networks and the Future of Global Governance* (Ottawa: IDRC Publishers, 2000), with Jim Whitman, "Global Governance as the Friendly Face of Unaccountable Power," *Security Dialogue* 33, no. 1 (2002): 45–57; Richter, "Public-Private Partnerships."

Chapter 5 considers the impact and potential of national policies that can support ongoing regional and global efforts by focusing on U.S. global health diplomacy. Putatively, supporting foreign capacity in infectious disease surveillance and response is a policy initiative that could promote U.S. security and welfare interests by building health cooperation in troubled regions of the world as a frontline defense against pandemics and both fostering regional stability and promoting American humanitarian values worldwide. In addition to the national security implications of disease control that President Obama most recently noted, U.S. Secretary of State Hillary Clinton captured the relationship between infectious disease and the promotion of human rights in a 2009 speech: "Basic levels of well-being—food, shelter, health, and education—and of common goods—like environmental sustainability, protection against pandemic disease, and provisions for refugees—are necessary for people to exercise their rights."[62] Chapter 5 investigates existing U.S. foreign policy initiatives in strengthening infectious disease surveillance and response abroad. The goal of that chapter is to better understand this particular aspect of U.S. global health diplomacy and to consider how it might best complement transnational efforts in infectious disease control while furthering U.S. security and humanitarian interests.

Chapter 6 summarizes the volume's conclusions and offers some suggestions for further research.

---

62. The White House, "Statement by the President on Global Health Initiative" (Washington, DC: Executive Office of the President, May 5, 2009); Hillary Rodham Clinton, "Remarks on Human Rights Agenda for the 21st Century" (speech, Georgetown University, Washington, DC, December 14, 2009).

2

CASES OF INTERNATIONAL COOPERATION

This chapter provides the empirical foundation for the theoretical discussion of interstate cooperation in chapter 3 and of transnational governance in chapter 4. After presenting the global architecture for infectious disease surveillance and response, it describes the origins, evolution, and operations of the Mekong Basin, Middle Eastern, and East African disease surveillance networks, and introduces a new international nongovernmental organization (INGO) designed to bring these three and other regional networks together to facilitate coordination among networks on a global scale.

The Messy World of Global Infectious Disease Surveillance and Response

Before considering the three networks, it is important to outline the larger global framework governing infectious disease surveillance.[1] Today the fight against infectious disease has brought together international governmental organizations, states, nongovernmental organizations, and private actors in an array of new initiatives. Forms of cooperation and governance structures have proliferated within this issue area—a policy space recently described as "pasture open for all."[2]

The proliferation of actors in international health governance is very recent, however. Over most of its history, the control over infectious diseases

---

1. The characterization comes from Mark W. Zacher and Tania J. Keefe, whose recent work concludes that global "health governance is complicated and messy." See *The Politics of Global Health Governance: United by Contagion* (New York: Palgrave Macmillan, 2008), 135.
2. David P. Fidler, "Reflections on the Revolution in Health and Foreign Policy," *Bulletin of the World Health Organization* 85, no. 3 (2007): 243–44.

has been the responsibility of states and intergovernmental organizations. Historically, international efforts to control infectious disease in peacetime date to the mid-nineteenth century: a period of rapidly growing industrialization, trade, and travel. The 1851 International Sanitary Conference in Paris constituted "the first attempt at international governance in infectious disease,"[3] largely through setting standards for quarantines, and was followed rapidly by several international conventions and institutions later subsumed under the League of Nations Health Organization (LNHO) in 1920.[4]

In 1948, the World Health Organization (WHO) succeeded the LNHO and assumed responsibility over existing international sanitary regulations. WHO organized itself into six regional offices and convenes its full membership annually at the World Health Assembly.[5] WHO also revised the sanitary regulations in 1951 and 1969, when they were retitled as international health regulations (IHR).[6] Because technological optimism concerning the control of infectious diseases was the prevailing sentiment until the 1980s, activities directed to the core functions of disease control—sophisticated surveillance for outbreaks, efficient emergency response for containment, and transboundary cooperation to stop or slow propagation—were minimal.

Before the mid-1990s, the IHR obligated governments to report outbreaks of only three diseases to WHO—plague, cholera, and yellow fever.[7] Reporting was irregular, however, because countries feared the economic consequences of reporting an outbreak or governments lacked information of outbreaks.

Beginning in the 1990s, the growth and diffusion of information and communication technologies and the worldwide emergence and reemergence of new and old infectious diseases began to fundamentally change this system in several ways. First, WHO reasserted itself as an active leader in global infectious disease. After much debate, in 2005, the 193 national members of the World Health Assembly concluded a revision of the IHR that set a new international standard for infectious disease surveillance and response. The new regulations are designed to protect populations world-

3.   WHO, "History of WHO and International Cooperation in Public Health," www.who.or.jp/GENERAL/history_wkc.html.

4.   Sandra J. MacLean, "Microbes, Mad Cows, and Militaries: Exploring the Links between Health and Security," *Security Dialogue* 39, no. 5 (2008): 479.

5.   The six regions are Africa, Southeast Asia, the Americas, the Eastern Mediterranean, Europe, and the Western Pacific. Membership in the World Health Assembly now includes 193 nations.

6.   Zacher and Keefe, *Politics of Global Health Governance*, 7.

7.   Cholera was the disease that prompted a global public health response as it spread from South Asia, to the Middle East, and then to Europe and the Americas in the first half of the nineteenth century. By the time of the first International Sanitary Conference in 1851, yellow fever and plague were also extant. These three diseases became the focus of international infectious disease regulation.

wide without interfering with travel and trade. Under the revised regulations, member states must notify the WHO Secretariat of "public health emergencies of international concern" (PHEICs), and better identify and respond to these events.[8] IHR 2005 broadened disease coverage from just three to more than fifteen, with the possibility of more, and required the reporting on other PHEICs such as incidents that involve the natural, accidental, or deliberate release of chemical, biological, or radiological materials. The new regulations formally permitted WHO to accept information on outbreaks from nongovernmental sources—a process that had begun de facto a decade earlier. WHO was also given new decision-making powers to create specific rules or guidelines with respect to emergency outbreaks and long-term problems—so-called emergency recommendations and standing recommendations. The regulations themselves constitute international legal obligations and the WHO Secretariat can encourage compliance by members with its recommendations through its power to name and shame. Member states, in turn, committed themselves to acquire the capabilities to gather and distribute information on diseases and to notify WHO and neighboring countries of all events potentially constituting a public health emergency, to maintain a national focal point to mediate communication between the government and WHO, and to comply with WHO response recommendations.[9] The IHR 2005 encouraged states to participate in regional surveillance networks to enhance their capabilities.[10] The requirements take effect beginning in 2007 and are to be verifiably effective on a global basis by 2012.

Currently, WHO's role is to "internationalize" a disease outbreak as a legitimate global concern; mobilize financial, technical, and human resources to respond to a large-scale outbreak; and provide advice and information to national public health ministries, the media, and the public. Ultimately, WHO is the necessary facilitator of international dialogue and the impresario needed to meet an outbreak of global importance. Because of its global reach, WHO carries a measure of credibility with the national health officials who request its involvement.

An organization like WHO faces certain constraints as well. WHO's established credentials can lead to suspicion that it represents the interests of its most powerful and wealthy members, who supply most of its supplemental funds. Also, by virtue of its recommendation power, WHO

---

8.   PHEICs are defined as extraordinary events that pose a public health risk through the international spread of disease to the rest of the world.

9.   Zacher and Keefe, *Politics of Global Health Governance*, 74.

10.   Section 44 of the IHR 2005. Philippe Calain, "From the Field Side of the Binoculars: A Different View on Global Public Health Surveillance," *Health Policy Planning* 22, no. 1 (2007): 13–20.

represents what might be called the outbreak police to those who question its authority to sanction nations. Its global reach and the vagaries of its regional structure can make it an awkward or oversized bureaucracy for addressing matters where small distances and short periods can have great consequences. Furthermore, its core budget is far less than is needed to fulfill its worldwide mandate.

A second change wrought by new technologies and diseases was the launch of many other global initiatives within and outside the WHO during the decade leading up to the IHR 2005. Very briefly, these include the following:

- WHO's Global Influenza Surveillance Network, which predates the modern era, but has expanded to include 126 national influenza centers in 88 countries that coordinate the analysis of data samples collected during influenza season, which is vital to the production of effective vaccines;
- WHO's Global Outbreak Alert and Response Network (GOARN) made up of more than 140 governments, NGOs, and multipartner health groups that exchange information and help coordinate response teams needed for the implementation of the IHR;
- Program for Monitoring Emerging Diseases (ProMED), an electronically linked group of health professionals that, since 1994, has communicated through the Internet on outbreaks of infectious diseases and acute exposure to toxins to more than 40,000 subscribers in more than 185 countries;
- Global Public Health Intelligence Network (GPHIN), which was co-created by the Canadian government and WHO in 1997 to monitor media sources worldwide for information on disease outbreaks, bioterrorism threats, and other natural and man-made disasters. After screening the information, GPHIN releases the data to its subscribers in real time;
- U.S. Department of Defense's Global Emerging Infectious Surveillance and Response System (GEIS), which maintains epidemiological laboratories (in Egypt, Kenya, Indonesia, Peru, and Thailand) that monitor infectious disease. These facilities coordinate information and research and report back to the main DOD-GEIS laboratories in the United States. Although the primary goal for the system is to monitor and prevent disease outbreaks that could affect military personnel, preventative measures extend to the local community to prevent the

spread of communicable diseases. It coordinates its projects with other international organizations to provide a more global network for disease response and surveillance. Chapter 5 offers a more extensive discussion of the GEIS program;

- World Animal Health Organization (OIE), which accepts information on animal diseases submitted officially by the agricultural authority of its 174 member states and 36 international organizations and NGOs; and
- One World, One Health initiative, launched jointly by the UN's Food and Agricultural Organization (FAO), OIE, WHO, the United Nations Children Fund (UNICEF), the World Bank, and the United Nations System Influenza Coordination (UNSIC). This strategic framework seeks to diminish the risk and minimize the impact of epidemics and pandemics by enhancing both human and animal disease intelligence, surveillance, and emergency response systems at national, regional, and international levels, with a particular emphasis at the national level.[11]

A third change in the policy environment was the emergence of several regional initiatives directed at infectious disease surveillance and control. For example, the Mekong Basin Disease Surveillance network works with the ASEAN nations[12] and the ASEAN +3 (China, Japan, and South Korea) to form pan-regional animal health centers and to establish networks in surveillance, diagnosis, and communications. More recently, ASEAN developed a regional strategy on highly pathogenic avian influenza that has led to information sharing about national practices among members. Beginning in 2007, ASEAN +3 began the Emerging Infectious Disease Program, which, along with ASEAN's Sectoral Group on Livestock, hopes to work with national and international actors to support regional coordination and partnerships between the public and animal health sectors,[13] and aspires to cooperation on a variety of related issues.[14]

---

11. *Contributing to One World, One Health: A Strategic Framework for Reducing the Risks of Infectious Diseases at the Animal-Human-Ecosystems Interface* (Rome: Food and Agriculture Organization, World Organization for Animal Health (OIE), World Health Organization, United Nations Influenza Coordination, United Nations Children's Fund (UNICEF), and the World Bank), www.fao.org/docrep/011/aj137e/aj137e00.htm; Food and Agriculture Organization, *Global Programme for the Prevention and Control of Highly Pathogenic Avian Influenza Report* (Rome: Food and Agriculture Organization, 2008), 10.

12. The members include Indonesia, Malaysia, the Philippines, Singapore, Thailand, Brunei, Burma (Myanmar), Cambodia, Laos, and Vietnam.

13. *Contributing to One World, One Health,* 14.

14. ASEAN Secretariat, "Joint Statement of the Third ASEAN PLUS Three Health Ministers Meeting" (meeting statement, ASEAN, Jakarta, Indonesia, 2008), www.aseanplus3-eid.info/newsread.php?nid=98&gid=3.

Finally, technological advances and diffusion of ICTs and the emergence and reemergence of infectious diseases coupled with a new global standard or norm for national policies embodied in IHR 2005 also led to an increase in funding and in the number of funding sources available for infectious disease control. For example, U.S. funding for global health has quintupled in the past decade. The rapid increase in spending on global public health by public and private actors brought a host of new nongovernmental actors into this issue area. These health NGOs, together with governments and international organizations, have created new public-private partnerships in the field of public health generally and in disease surveillance and response in particular.

The Mekong Basin Disease Surveillance network, the Middle East Consortium on Infectious Disease, and the East African Integrated Disease Surveillance Network are three of these public-private partnerships. Each is described in the following sections.

The Mekong Basin Disease Surveillance Network

MBDS member countries share land and water borders crossed daily by thousands of people and animals, making control of communicable disease a long-standing challenge. Growing interdependence in the region and the rise of novel, highly communicable diseases, many of zoonotic origin, emphasized rapid identification of the type and source of infections, vaccine development, and treatment regimens.[15]

Beginning informally at a meeting in Bangkok in 1999, health ministries from the six MBDS partner countries, along with epidemiologists and other specialists, began working together to share information and biological samples on disease outbreaks and to develop the capacity to control communicable diseases, especially among marginalized populations. With the support and encouragement of the Rockefeller Foundation, the initial activities of MBDS included regular cross-border information exchange at border sites, training health workers in epidemiology and disease surveillance and response techniques, and planning for joint outbreak investigation and response.

By late 2001, cooperation had progressed to the point where the ministers of health of the six member countries signed a simple memorandum of understanding. The document recognized their many existing coopera-

---

15.   Ann Marie Kimball et al., "Regional Infectious Disease Surveillance Networks and Their Potential to Facilitate the Implementation of the International Health Regulations," *Medical Clinics North America* 92 (2008): 1459–71.

tive efforts and aimed specifically at strengthening national and subregional capabilities in disease surveillance and outbreak response with regard to five priority diseases.[16] The understanding contemplated information exchange, cooperative systems development, human resource development, and joint outbreak response.[17] The agreement had a life span of five years.

A new memorandum of understanding (MOU) signed by MBDS health ministers in May 2007 continued the organization for an indefinite period. The Guangxi Zhuang Autonomous Region of the People's Republic of China became a member of MBDS in February 2008. The 2007 memorandum expands the network's aims to monitor and control a wider range of priority diseases and public health emergencies of international concern. The 2007 MOU calls for sharing information essential to developing health and social policy that will reduce the burdens arising from these priority diseases.[18] The new memorandum also called on members to create a six-year action plan to go into effect in January 2008. The expanded agenda was driven in part by new global norms and responsibilities established under the World Health Organization's IHR 2005.

The general objectives of MBDS included the development of mechanisms for strong cross-border programs implemented initially at five pilot sites that would grow to thirty-seven by 2009. Cross-border cooperation especially at key points of entry is especially useful in monitoring and rapidly responding to a problem before it becomes a global threat.[19] Data from routine surveillance on priority diseases at each site is exchanged through national coordinators and adjacent province site coordinators. Reports of suspected outbreaks are also conveyed when detected. Information exchanges are carried out daily, weekly, monthly, or quarterly at the various sites. Improved Internet connectivity within and between member states and technical training programs have enhanced communications, but standardization issues remain.[20]

---

16. The initial priority diseases were dengue infection, malaria, severe diarrhea (including cholera), vaccine preventable diseases, and other diseases with subregional significance. See Mekong Basin Disease Surveillance Cooperation (MBDSC), "Memorandum of Understanding Among the Health Ministries of the Six Mekong Countries on the Mekong Basin Disease Surveillance (MBDS) Project" (memorandum, Nonthaburi, Thailand: MBDSC, 2001).

17. MBDSC, "Memorandum of Understanding."

18. Priority diseases now include severe acute respiratory syndrome (SARS), avian influenza, malaria, dengue, human immunodeficiency virus (HIV), cholera, acute flaccid paralysis (AFP), typhoid, measles, and tuberculosis (TB). See MBDSC, "The Extension of Memorandum of Understanding among the Health Ministries of the Six Mekong Countries on the Mekong Basin Disease Surveillance (MBDS) Project" (memorandum, Nonthaburi, Thailand: MBDSC, 2007).

19. Nkuchia M. M'ikanatha et al., ed., *Infectious Disease and Surveillance* (Malden, MA: Blackwell Publishing, 2007).

20. Kimball et al., "Regional Infectious Disease," 1459–71.

By 2006, MBDS partners had established joint outbreak investigation and response capability through the creation of cross-border teams made up of health, customs, immigration, and border officials. These teams have already investigated and contained dengue fever outbreaks between Laos and Thailand provincial sites, a typhoid outbreak between provincial sites in Laos and Vietnam, and an avian flu incident in Laos after detecting an infected Laotian citizen in Thailand.

Human capacity building through the training of healthcare personnel is another important function of MBDS. The joint Thai-U.S. Centers for Disease Control and Prevention (CDC) Field Epidemiology Training Program, Mahidol University, and Southeast Asian Ministers of Education-TropMed Organization conduct annual training for frontline and supervisory public health officials. Participants receive skill enhancement in research, outbreak investigation, and communication, and establish working relations with officers from adjunct provinces in neighboring states. MBDS is currently enhancing training and capacity in field epidemiology through a regional Southeast Asian network—The International Group for Epidemiology and Response (TIGER)—and providing formal degree programs for veterinary and epidemiology professionals through distance learning with partners in the United States and Europe. MBDS has also linked with ProMED-mail to provide an integrated Internet-based reporting system for the region that will enable early warning of infectious diseases at all levels of the public health infrastructure of the member states.

To develop a more integrated approach to a possible pandemic influenza outbreak, each member state, and all six member states together, conducted tabletop simulation exercises in early 2007. Working with gaming and simulation experts from the RAND Corporation, this exercise was designed to foster cooperation and to identify weaknesses in detecting, monitoring, and tracking a highly infectious disease. This diagnostic tool is part of an ongoing MBDS initiative to monitor and assess the network's operations using agreed indicators and to make plans for coordinated policy response to emergencies.

Uniting these activities and programs means building trust, common practice, teamwork, and understanding among key personnel in the six states. Gradually, the organization's authority and legitimacy grew from its expertise and commitment, localized knowledge, timely and reliable information, and personal communication network, which allowed it to act quickly and effectively in an issue area where time is often of the essence. In governance terms, MBDS began and remains a direct action network rather than an

Figure 1. Cross-Border Cooperation in Relation to Other Core Strategies

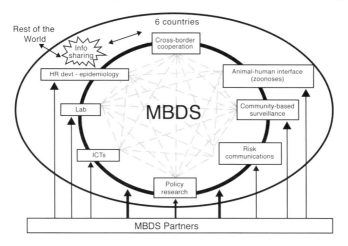

Source: MBDSC, Action Plan (2008–13)

advocacy network. It is not primarily concerned with consciousness raising or setting national or international agendas. Instead it acts in a well-defined policy niche with health officials and leaders from the community or provincial level across borders.

Between 2008 and 2013, the focus of MBDS partners is on implementing seven interrelated core strategies identified by MBDS leadership (see figure 1). These strategies include the following elements:

- maintaining and expanding cross-border cooperation,
- improving human-animal sector interface and strengthening community-based surveillance,
- strengthening epidemiology capacity,
- strengthening information and communications technologies (ICT) capacity,
- expanding laboratory capacity,
- improving risk communications, and
- conducting and applying policy research.[21]

Each strategy has a project leader from a different MBDS country and a steering committee with representatives from each member state. For example, Thailand will take the lead on lab capacity and epidemiological training, and Cambodia will assume a leadership role in community surveillance policies and procedures. This initiative represents an expansion

---

21. MBDSC, *Action Plan (2008–2013)* (Nonthaburi, Thailand: MBDSC, 2008).

Figure 2. MBDS Coordinating Mechanism

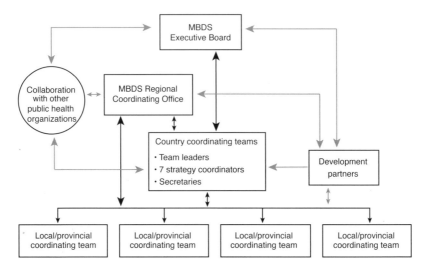

Source: MBDSC, Action Plan (2008–13)

and formalization of MBDS programs and may create greater complexity in coordinating with other regional and global actors engaged in these issues.

Since 2001, an executive board (EB) of the key policymakers of the six partners—typically, the senior public health directors who report directly to their respective health minister—has governed MBDS. The chairmanship of the board rotates to a different partner in successive years. The EB is assisted by the Coordinating Committee, that is, the contact persons assigned by the partners in charge of implementing and following up on regular activities. In 2006, the members created a permanent coordination site in Thailand located in the national health compound in Bangkok. MBDS interfaces with the members' national public health systems, which vary organizationally within each member state. Each public health director represented at MBDS can speak and act authoritatively on behalf of its own minister of health, however.

Partner organizations include the Rockefeller Foundation (which provided start-up and sustained funding), the Global Health and Security Initiative (GHSI) of the Nuclear Threat Initiative[22] (an American NGO

---

22. The Global Health and Security Initiative (GHSI) advocates threat reduction solutions, raises public awareness, and undertakes direct action projects that demonstrate innovative ways to reduce threats. For additional information, see the Global Health and Security Initiative Web site, www.ghsi.org.

that has orchestrated financial and technical support for the organization), Google.org (an ICT supporter), RAND (as trainers in pandemic response), WHO, United Nations System Influenza Coordination, Asian Development Bank, the Association of Southeast Asian Nations, and others (see figure 2).

MBDS's immediate challenges include sustaining its funding and effectively institutionalizing and assessing its programs. Funding is complicated by the multiple aims of donors and by international sanctions on Myanmar that bar it from receiving support from certain entities. Funders' aims vary: some are interested in MBDS per se, others are focused on a particular functional aspect of MBDS's operation (such as ICT infrastructure), some are focused on particular sectors (animal health, for example), and others are concerned with a particular disease (such as influenza). Although MBDS has benefited from long-standing supporters, the Rockefeller Foundation and the GHSI of the Nuclear Threat Initiative in particular, the various funder priorities make it more difficult for MBDS members to maintain control of the policy agenda. Sanctions placed on Myanmar also complicate operations. MBDS members laud Myanmar for its commitment to the organization, but it is nonetheless walled off from certain donors. Sustaining funding for MBDS operations is a concern, especially during periods of economic difficulty. MBDS, with the encouragement of some of its senior supporters, is drafting a master plan to anticipate and meet its long-term funding needs.

Increasingly, MBDS also faces the challenges of institutionalization and assessment. Initially, MBDS goals were not so much a specific health milestone or metric as creating a trusted network. Although this network is the backbone of the organization and indispensable to its effectiveness, it is also slow to develop and difficult to quantify to external funders. As its programs grow, along with greater coordination in budgetary planning, MBDS will likely need to strengthen its programmatic assessment activities and develop more explicit institutional rules and procedures.[23]

MBDS has also fostered some functional cooperation in policy domains related to infectious disease control. It can point to evidence of functional spillover in disaster relief cooperation. Immediately after Cyclone Nargis struck Myanmar in 2008, MBDS coordinated deployment of a rapid response team to assist refugees in the Myuangmya region (about fifty miles from the storm's center). Health workers from other MBDS countries, working on a bilateral basis, monitored outbreaks of infectious respiratory diseases

---

23. As of 2010, the Rockefeller Foundation had launched a programmatic review of its support for MBDS as part of a larger assessment of its grants in this area of public health.

and addressed other endemic diseases, such as cholera, and mosquito-borne diseases, such as malaria and dengue fever. Thanks to existing relationships and collaborative procedures it had developed, MBDS helped these teams access the region without the political delays that some multilateral initiatives faced. In addition to emergency response, because MBDS regularly convenes customs and commercial officials at community and provincial levels across borders, it serves as a forum and model for potential cooperation in expanded trade and tourism. Some believe that MBDS shies away from political controversy, however, and avoids expanding its efforts where the interests among its members diverge. MBDS officials concede that they were not successful in cooperating on intellectual property matters related to sharing prescription drugs because of political differences. Likewise, external critics believe that MBDS should do more in tracking migrant and mobile populations in the region, which can create special public health risks such as outbreak proneness or drug resistance, but that it has not tackled this challenge because of a lack of political will or technical capacity.[24] For the most part, MBDS has not led to the creation of supranational institutions as neofunctionalists might hope. It does, however, coordinate with larger regional and global actors as discussed. In addition, MBDS recently joined an initiative known as CHORDS (Connecting Health Organizations for Regional Disease Surveillance), which was inaugurated in April 2009 to knit together and share best practices among similar subregional infectious disease networks. CHORDS is discussed later in this chapter.

Middle East Consortium on Infectious Disease Surveillance

The Middle East Consortium on Infectious Disease Surveillance (MECIDS) was launched in November 2002 based on the recommendations made by Middle Eastern health and medical professionals participating in a meeting in Istanbul on regional cooperation on disease surveillance hosted by Search for Common Ground (SFCG).[25] Reflecting the mood at the meeting, an Israeli participant described it as "more than exciting." A Palestinian scientist added, "I expected more difficulty in finding common ground. People were

---

24. Personal interview, Bangkok, Thailand, April 6–10, 2009.
25. Search for Common Ground is an international nonprofit organization. It was founded in 1982 and works to transform the way the world deals with conflict. Its goal is to move the world away from adversarial approaches and toward collaborative problem solving. It uses media production (radio, TV, film, and print), mediation and facilitation, training, community organizing, sports, drama, and music to attempt to bring conflicting sides together to peacefully resolve issues. It is currently working in seventeen countries and has two main offices, in Washington, DC, and Brussels, Belgium. See www.sfcg.org.

professionals around the table. We are one epidemiological family. We are brothers and sisters in blood."[26]

Although the November 2002 meeting marked the official launch of MECIDS, SFCG and the Global Health and Security Initiative of the Nuclear Threat Initiative—a conflict resolution and a security NGO respectively—had laid the groundwork long before. SFCG had an established record of initiating track II dialogues on security and conflict issues in the Middle East. Working with NTI, its efforts were intensified with the heightened security concerns following the attacks on the United States on September 11, 2001. For these NGOs, the prevailing concern was on the potential for the proliferation of weapons of mass destruction to nonstate actors and the possibility of catastrophic terrorism, coupled with a sense of urgency to instigate some form of cooperative dialogue in the Middle East. Because of their interest in bioweapons, the search for partners led the two NGOs to the health ministries of governments in the region, and in turn to public health officials within the health ministries. The public health officials proved receptive to the possibility of establishing a regional dialogue because they had clear interests and responsibilities in transnational disease control and response, a problem that paralleled biosecurity and for which the solutions might prove similar.[27]

With this as its generative context, MECIDS's vision was to promote long-term health, stability, and security in the region. Participants agreed to cooperate for the twin aims of reducing the region's vulnerability to disease outbreaks, whether natural or caused by a biological weapon, and of providing ways for health professionals to build trust and confidence across national lines.[28] For example, the director of Jordan's Center for Disease Control and Israel's director of public health met for the first time under MECIDS auspices at a gathering held in Brussels in 2003, thus creating a critical link for coping with future regional problems in health.[29]

MECIDS members and partner organizations come from governments, universities, and nongovernmental organizations. Members include the public health directors of Jordan, Israel, and the Palestinian Authority; the

26. Middle East Consortium on Infectious Disease Surveillance (MECIDS), "Infectious Disease Surveillance: Middle East Regional Cooperation" (online report, Istanbul, Turkey, October 31–November 2, 2002), www.mecids.org.

27. Personal interview, Washington, DC, October 13, 2009.

28. MECIDS, "Infectious Disease Surveillance." Diseases of immediate concern included food-borne diseases, blood-borne diseases, and influenza-like diseases.

29. MECIDS, "Plenary Meeting Report" (meeting report, Brussels, Belgium, March 6–8, 2003), www.mecids.org/reports.php.

Cooperative Monitoring Center (CMC) at Amman, Jordan;[30] Tel Aviv University (Israel), and Al Quds University (Palestinian University in Jerusalem). Advisors include WHO (which works closely with the Palestinian community in Gaza), American and European NGOs, foreign governments, and private corporations. The Middle East Program of SFCG initially provided day-to-day management and coordination assistance. The GHSI of the Nuclear Threat Initiative (NTI) coordinates essential financial, material, and technical support.[31] The partners also hope to engage other countries in the region with a view to membership. Egypt has attended meetings as an observer.[32] No formal agreement or MOU supports the creation of MECIDS. MECIDS was and remains an informal organization held together by the good will of its members and partners.

MECIDS specific operational goals include the following:

- building the region's capacity in infectious diseases surveillance (especially helping their Palestinian colleagues build capable systems);[33]
- reducing the region's vulnerability to infectious diseases;
- facilitating interregional scientific cooperation; and
- standardizing methods for collecting, managing, reporting, and disseminating data and information among the members.[34]

MECIDS programs are designed to both improve each country's health systems and standardize health practices across the three nations.

Over the last several years, MECIDS has built an infrastructure to help Israel, Jordan, and the Palestinian Authority cooperate in detecting and managing disease outbreak. MECIDS members have identified and secured several immediate goals, which include meeting critical laboratory needs for species characterization and information sharing capacity, finalizing a common plan of action on avian influenza, and writing and implementing pandemic influenza cooperation procedures in accord with the World Health Assembly's 2005 International Health Regulation. MECIDS has

---

30. The Cooperative Monitoring Center at Amman (CMC) acts as a hub for collecting and sharing the MECIDS health data between participation countries. Officially inaugurated on October 16, 2003, the CMC seeks to promote the development of regional cooperative security issues through technology. In addition to public health, it focuses on border security, arms control and nonproliferation, and environmental security.

31. NTI is a U.S. nonprofit organization founded in 2001 by Ted Turner and Sam Nunn. NTI aims to strengthen global security by reducing the spread of nuclear, biological, and chemical weapons, and also to reduce the risk that they will actually be used. See "About NTI," www.nti.org.

32. See "MECIDS: Members and Partners," www.mecids.org/members.php.

33. In fact, Israeli laboratories have donated supplies and training to the Palestinian Central Public Health Laboratories in Amman.

34. See the MECIDS Web site, www.mecids.org.

also made substantial progress on longer-term goals, including pursuing epidemiological, laboratory, and computer training; creating joint research opportunities; improving the level of communication among health professionals in the three jurisdictions; and ensuring financial stability and sustainability of MECIDS.

The consortium's initial project was to develop and enhance a food-borne disease surveillance system in Israel, Jordan, and the Palestinian territories based on a joint initiative that monitored such diseases for six months in East Jerusalem, West Jerusalem, and a Jordanian city.[35] With advice from Sandia National Laboratories, MECIDS established a Web site to routinely share data about the incidence of particular diseases such as salmonella and shigellosis and they agreed on procedures for communicating in the case of an outbreak that threatens their populations. As part of this effort, MECIDS launched an interventional field epidemiology course. In collaboration with the European Program for Intervention Epidemiology Training (EPIET), it conducted the first regional epidemiological training course for Middle Eastern public health professionals from the three nations in September 2004. In 2005, when avian influenza reached the Mediterranean region, and along with it fears that the disease could infect humans, the region's ability to deal with a human influenza pandemic climbed higher on the list of MECIDS's priorities.

Beginning in 2005, MECIDS built an infrastructure in the region to help nations cooperate in managing disease outbreaks including avian influenza.[36] Alex Leventhal, director of Israel's Health Ministry Department of International Relations and a MECIDS principal, explained the rationale for expanding the organization's agenda: "We decided to take the infrastructure of MECIDS, with its people and friendships, to meet the growing health needs of the region."[37] Over the next three years, MECIDS partners went on both to develop individual national plans and a collective plan for a regional flu pandemic and to test these plans individually and together using tabletop simulations.[38] When swine flu cases were identified in May 2009, MECIDS

---

35. The project included three components: the creation of sentinel clinics to identify pathogenic agents; the registration of key data about all hospitalized patients; and the conducting of a population prevalence study. MECIDS, "Plenary Meeting Report."

36. MECIDS, "First Four-Way Meeting on 'Bird Flu': Palestinians, Jordanians, and Egyptians Coordinate on Avian Influenza Risk" (meeting report, Istanbul, Turkey, December 11–14, 2005), www.mecids.org.

37. Karin Kloosterman, "Israel, PA and Jordan Cooperate as Flu Threat Grows," *Common Ground News Service,* May 2005, www.commongroundnews.org/article.php?id=25446&an=en&sp=0.

38. Following WHO guidelines, MECIDS members made plans to strengthen cooperation in the following areas: planning and coordination, situation monitoring and assessment, prevention and containment, health system response, and communications. MECIDS, "First Four-Way Meeting on 'Bird Flu.'"

officials met immediately to jointly implement the pandemic plan, including matters related to risk communication to their populations.[39]

MECIDS members convene several times a year to update each other on recent developments in the health field, to renew their acquaintances, and to plan future activities. At the annual MECIDS conference in January 2007, members took an important step toward transitioning to a self-sustaining consortium run by MECIDS members. During this meeting, they agreed on a new governance structure, elected a MECIDS executive chairperson, and formed an executive board to replace a more informal steering committee.[40] SFCG continues to provide staff support to MECIDS, including a secretariat based in East Jerusalem that facilitates communication among consortium members, sets and monitors deadlines for action, and performs other administrative functions as needed. Previously, SFCG and professional facilitators had played a more extensive role in creating modalities for steering committee meetings.

As currently constituted, the day-to-day operation of MECIDS includes the following activities:

- Regular, cross-border information exchanges. Early on, MECIDS members agreed that regional cooperation and communication on a regular basis would improve response to disease outbreaks. Agreeing on the need for regional cooperation on sharing information and laboratory data, each country submits its data on the tenth of every month to the MECIDS program associate and then onward to be distributed to all members in the form of a newsletter and harmonized data form from the CMC in Amman.[41]

- Targeted efforts on food- and water-borne diseases and other biological threats. As noted, MECIDS members initially identified food-borne disease as a priority concern and established a disease surveillance system compromised of a network of laboratories for identifying disease outbreaks. MECIDS members have established protocols for specimen collection and diagnosis of diarrheal illness to assess food-borne disease in the region and to create a mechanism for identifying potential infectious disease outbreaks due to common food products. Members send their data routinely to one another, opening the lines of communication

---

39. Personal interview, Washington, DC, May 26, 2009.

40. MECIDS, "Middle East Consortium on Infectious Disease Surveillance Meeting" (meeting report, Amman, Jordan, January 16–18, 2007), www.medcids.org/reports.php.

41. MECIDS, "The Middle East Consortium on Infectious Disease Surveillance" (meeting report, Istanbul, Turkey, June 15–18, 2005), www.mecids.org.

between the departments of public health in each entity, and have been instrumental in detecting two significant outbreaks, salmonella and mumps, providing evidence that the system is functioning properly.[42] When avian influenza emerged in the region in 2005, MECIDS demonstrated itself to be an important channel for rapid communication in responding to the most pressing threats facing the region.

- Monthly executive council meetings. MECIDS Executive Council members meet regularly to discuss specific issues such as cross-border coordination, review their regional influenza preparedness plan, consult on emerging influenza cases, and maintain a close working relationship among people responsible for infectious disease detection and response. To the extent that political tensions limit travel in the region, the group meets by conference call.

- Regional scientific council meetings. The human and animal sectors from Jordan, Israel, and the Palestinian Authority have met with experts from the WHO and other invited technical experts to review the recently completed regional pandemic preparedness plan and to put a common plan of action into place. Regional conferences allow the regional plan to be examined with regard to risk communication, vaccine policy, cross-border transport, training, and applied research. Because the plan includes issues related to livestock and migratory animals, coordination with agricultural ministries in monitoring and culling potentially infected animal populations is necessary. In November 2007, the MECIDS partners invited WHO representatives to conduct a workshop on IHR 2005. Israel and Jordan are WHO members and legally bound by the regulations. The Palestinian authority participated as a WHO nonmember. In 2008, Jordanian, Israeli, and Palestinian health and agriculture experts recommended that their governments adopt principles and procedures for common action during outbreaks of avian and other potential pandemic influenza.[43]

---

42. Alex Levanthal and Dany Cohen, "Surveillance Systems in Practice" (presentation, International Meeting on Emerging Disease and Response 2009, Vienna, Austria, February 15, 2009), www.imed.isid.org/IMED2009/preliminary_schedule.shtml.

43. The principles include ongoing consultation among the Palestinian, Jordanian, and Israeli health and agriculture ministries at all levels in the area of avian influenza; rapid communication among all three any time there is suspicion of a case; if the Protection Zone and the Surveillance Zone do not cross a boundary, nations should inform each other of any procedures they plan to employ that deviate from existing national plans; nations should consult with each other before taking a decision to vaccinate poultry; all partners should have enough resources to implement necessary, agreed control measures; all partners should assess the situation, evaluate their needs, and if they have gaps, should, together, appeal for international assistance; in addition to consulting about emerging events, partners should share post-event reports in order to facilitate learning. MECIDS, "Avian and Pandemic Influenza Sub-Regional Common Plan of Action" (online report), www.mecids.org/reports.php.

- Laboratory and risk communication training. WHO's guidance on avian and pandemic influenza recommends that countries receive training in laboratory methods needed for H5N1 diagnosis, epidemiological investigation, and risk communication. MECIDS workshops on these topics have provided this knowledge with the added value of training in interpersonal communication and cooperative problem solving.
- Informatics and equipment. With the support of IBM, MECIDS has installed an innovative data-sharing network for the MECIDS partners, known as the Public Health Information Affinity Domain (PHIAD). This system is the first on-demand one in the public health industry, enabling the integration and sharing of data generated at clinical and public health institutions across proprietary systems and political boundaries.[44] Installation of the new system in 2008 included the supply of computers and servers as well as training for those who will be handling the epidemiological surveillance data, first at a national level, and then at a regional level for the sharing of information among partner countries.[45] Private companies are also supporting capacity building by donating critical laboratory equipment. In particular, the partners are engaging with PulseNet[46] Middle East for the supply of pulsed field gel electrophoresis (PFGE) equipment and associated training, which allow for timely and procedurally uniform identification of infectious disease strains.

The GHSI has provided essential financial and technical support to MECIDS. The World Bank has provided MECIDS with a grant that will

44. The system is built on international coding systems, as well as the coordination between open-source technologies and the Integrating the Healthcare Enterprise (IHE) initiative in the use of standards to allow multinational public health reporting and surveillance. PHIAD supports hierarchical data flow across domains. Each regional PHIAD collects data from local sources, such as doctors and veterinarians. The regional PHIAD then forwards appropriate information to a national PHIAD, which is administered by a disease control organization such as the Centers for Disease Control and Prevention (CDC). PHIAD can extend this hierarchy of data sharing to international partnerships. At each level, different data-sharing policies concerning person identification, location identification, authorship, and results can be implemented. The ability to share public health data electronically paves the way for sophisticated and advanced analysis tools that visualize the population's health, detect outbreaks, determine the effectiveness of policy, and perform forecast modeling. See the AlphaWorks Services: Public Health Information Affinity Domain (PHIAD) Web site, http://services.alphaworks. ibm.com/phiad/.

45. MECIDS, "MECIDS Partners Consider Cooperation with BM Research and the Consortium's Strategic Direction" (meeting report, Allenby/King Hussein Bridge, June 19–20, 2006), www.mecids.org.

46. PulseNet is a national network of public health and food regulatory agency laboratories coordinated by the U.S. Centers for Disease Control and Prevention (CDC). The network consists of state health departments, local health departments, and federal agencies (CDC, USDA/FSIS, FDA). See the CDC PulseNet Web site, www.cdc.gov/PULSEnet/.

allow the members to strengthen laboratory and secretarial capacity. As a result, MECIDS is now a self-governing body run by the MECIDS members. Other financial supporters are the Global Opportunity Fund (a governmental organization the United Kingdom) and the Gates Foundation. Becton Dickinson and Company has donated a three-year supply of reagents and other medical supplies needed for laboratory diagnosis, and, as noted, IBM has made in-kind donations that included the development of a new, innovative approach to handling epidemiological data through a shared information network for the MECIDS partners.

Given the sensitive political circumstances of the region, equity is a fundamental principle governing the consortium's transition to a self-sustaining entity. The governance of MECIDS is based on an executive council composed of an executive chairperson and executive board, supported by national MECIDS coordinators and a secretariat. Each member country holds the position of the chairperson for a year on a rotating basis allowing each MECIDS party an opportunity to fill this position. Alex Leventhal, director of Israel's Health Ministry's Department of International Relations and the consortium's first chairperson underscored this point: "The idea behind MECIDS is that everybody is equal."[47] The executive board comprises three members from each participating country, one of which must be a senior public health official from the participating Ministry of Health. The other team members are the laboratory supervisor and the country coordinator who liaises with the secretariat. The key decision-making norm of the executive board is consensus. Absent consensus among all members, decisions do not proceed. Executive board decisions are reviewed and evaluated at subsequent meetings. The country coordinators and the secretariat are the professional staff that handles most of the day-to-day tasks, including data sharing, meeting and function logistics, and documenting progress. The secretariat has two locations: operations are conducted from East Jerusalem, where the coordinator sits in the offices of SFCG; data handling, analytics, and board meetings are handled from Amman at the CMC on the campus of the Royal Scientific Society of Jordan.

In addition to political sensitivities in the region and the logistical challenges they can present to MECIDS as a transnational body, challenges include information security, coordination between animal and human health sectors, poverty, particularly among the Palestinian population, and long-

---

47. Dale Gavlak, "Catching Outbreaks Wherever They Occur," *World Health Organization Bulletin* 87, no. 10 (October 2009), who.int/bulletin/volumes/87/10/09-031009/en/.

term sustainability through financial support, human resource investment, and strategic planning.[48]

Despite these challenges, MECIDS's accomplishments are substantial. First, the relationships built through it have extended into a real-time communication network essential to emergency response. Second, the integrated surveillance system for food- and water-borne diseases has translated into surveillance for other infectious diseases of public health importance, such as tuberculosis or avian influenza. Since the recent cases of avian influenza emerged in the region, MECIDS has proved to be an important channel for rapid communication in responding to the most pressing threats facing the region. Potentially, such a network may be critical for early recognition and response should there be a deliberate attack using a biological agent to cause disease. In a region already deeply troubled by acts of terrorism, such an attack is a very real concern.

MECIDS hopes to continue to strengthen the ability to detect, characterize, and analyze infectious disease at every level in the participating nations, and to enhance mechanisms for sharing information across borders. Although it is communicated sotto voce, MECIDS members hope that the cooperation and confidence building associated with this project might give rise to cooperation on other issues, moving the region closer to peace. Members and partners also hope that MECIDS will serve as a model for creating infectious disease surveillance networks in other regions of the world. The principals stress, however, that they do not address political issues directly and do believe that this stance facilitates their institutional effectiveness in coping with factional divisions within their home governments. Assad Ramlawi, the Palestinian Authority Ministry's director of primary care and public health and a MECIDS Executive Board member captured this sentiment: "Political tensions are one issue and disease intervention is another."[49]

MECIDS has to date not led to functional spillover into divergent policy areas. Members have expanded their remit in the area of infectious disease and hope to share lessons learned in areas of chronic disease prevention and treatment by their respective health ministries in the future. As noted, the emerging preparedness plans established under MECIDS for coping with infectious disease pandemic and the network of trusted individuals MECIDS members have nurtured strengthens national and regional emer-

---

48. See Global Health Security Initiative, "Projects: Middle East Consortium in Infectious Disease Surveillance," www.ghsi.org/projects/mecids.html.
49. Gavlak, "Catching Outbreaks."

gency preparedness policies and capacities generally. Finally, MECIDS members note that theirs is not an exclusive club and that they could expand membership to other countries in the region.

East Africa Integrated Disease Surveillance Network

In February 2000, at a meeting called by the Tanzanian National Institute of Medical Research (NIMR),[50] the health ministries of Kenya, Tanzania, and Uganda, along with national health research and academic institutions from those three nations, collectively founded the East African Integrated Disease Surveillance Network (EAIDSNet).[51] They created the network to improve the quality of available data on communicable diseases and to increase the flow of information among participants to improve the health of the region's population through strengthening epidemic preparedness and response. Ultimately, EAIDSNet hoped to reduce morbidity and mortality from common communicable diseases by establishing a strong regional network capable of generating useful epidemiological information for early warning of impending epidemics. The network also intended to support joint planning and the implementation of disease control measures.[52]

The creation of EAIDSNet was inspired, in part, by the treaty to establish the East African Community (EAC), signed by Tanzania, Uganda, and Kenya in November 1999 and ratified the following year.[53] The EAC is a regional intergovernmental organization, headquartered in Arusha, Tanzania, with the aim of widening and deepening cooperation among partner states in political, economic, and social fields for their mutual benefit. The initial EAC countries established a customs union in 2005 and the five member states (which now include Rwanda and Burundi) are working toward establishing a common market in 2010, a monetary union by 2012, and ulti-

---

50. The Tanzania National Institute for Medical Research (NIMR) is a parastatal service organization under the Ministry of Health established after the demise of the first East African Community in 1977. In 1979, the NIMR was directed by the Tanzanian parliament to take over all health research institutions in the country that previously fell under the auspices of the defunct East African Medical Research Council.

51. The main Tanzanian collaborators included the National Institute for Medical Research, Ministry of Health, Ministry of Health and Social Welfare, Public Health Association, and School of Public Health and Social Sciences of Muhimbili University. The Ugandan participants included the Ministry of Health, National Health Research Organization, and Institute of Public Health of Makerere University. The Kenyan representatives included the Ministry of Health, Medical Research Institute, National Health Research and Development Center, and School of Public Health of Moi University.

52. East African Community, "Treaty for the Establishment of the East African Community" (October 7, 2009), www.eac.int.

53. Rwanda and Burundi became full members of the community on July 1, 2007.

mately a political federation of the East African states.[54] Article 118 of the treaty outlines future cooperation in health activities between partner states in health delivery systems, pharmaceutical policies, national health policies and legislation, research and development, training, and illegal drug policies. Significantly, the treaty specifies the need to take joint action towards the prevention and control of communicable and noncommunicable diseases and to control pandemics and epidemics of communicable and vector-borne diseases such as HIV/AIDS, cholera, malaria, hepatitis, and yellow fever that might endanger the health and welfare of the residents of partner states. The treaty also urges cooperation between partner states in facilitating mass immunization and other public health community campaigns.[55]

The EAC and EAIDSNet also drew inspiration from a long, if uneven, history of intergovernmental cooperation in East Africa and substantial collaboration in medical and scientific education and practice.[56] One observer described regional cooperation in health as "normal" and a likely foundation for improved regional relations.[57]

The resulting organization was launched with financial assistance from the Rockefeller Foundation of New York. The Rockefeller Foundation had long been active both in East Africa and in public health. Drawing on its experience in the region and analogous efforts in infectious disease control in Southeast Asia, the foundation made several grants to the health ministries of each founding member of EAIDSNet, to university and research organizations in the region, and in support of the activities of an EAIDSNet Secretariat housed in Dar es Salaam.[58] Although fully consistent with the vision articulated in the EAC treaty, EAIDSNet was not formally part of the community during its initial years.

During its first two years of operation, EAIDSNet established the following specific objectives:

---

54. See the East African Community Portal, December 27, 2009, www.eac.int.
55. East African Community, "Treaty for the Establishment of the East African Community."
56. Kenya, Tanzania, and Uganda have a history of cooperation as partners in several regional arrangements over the course of the last century. Kenya and Uganda founded a customs union in 1917, with Tanganyika joining in 1927. An East African High Commission existed between 1948 and 1961, an East African Common Services Organization from 1961 to 1967, the first East African Community from 1967 to 1977, and an East African Cooperation initiative from 1993 to 2000 (www.eac.int/component/content/article/34-body-text-area/70-establishment-eaidsnet.html). In medicine and science, the three countries historically coordinated in recognizing medical credentials and in education, with Makerere University serving as a common educational affiliation for many in the region. In infectious diseases, the three countries had worked together to form a common plan to address malaria outbreaks immediately prior to the creation of EAIDSNet. Personal interview, Atlanta, GA, December 18, 2009; Washington, DC, November 25, 2009.
57. Personal interview, Atlanta, GA, December 18, 2009.
58. Personal interview, December 18, 2009; Personal interview, Atlanta, GA, December 22, 2009.

- developing and strengthening appropriate communication channels within and between the East African Partner States to facilitate integrated disease surveillance and response (IDSR) and disease control efforts;
- providing effective information for planning and decision-making using various tools such as computerized geographical information systems;
- ensuring continuous exchange of information, expertise, and advocacy for disease surveillance and control activities in the region through different forums;
- promoting the exchange and dissemination of relevant information on IDSR and other disease control activities for policymaking;
- developing strategies for minimizing the risk and effect of disease transmission within the region; and
- strengthening capacities for implementation of disease surveillance and control activities.[59]

Members recognized that meeting these goals would require strengthening national disease surveillance systems, identifying priority diseases, improving border district capacities at key regional transit points, enhancing joint response capability, incorporating new techniques and technologies, and coordinating with the larger integration effort in East Africa.[60]

The initiative was, by most accounts, "slow in getting going," because the organization emphasized collective agenda-setting by the membership rather than one imposed by an external donor or international organization.[61] Over the course of its first four years, however, the network made progress on several of its goals. In addition to strengthening the IDSR activities of each member state, it established a thirteen-member steering committee and a three-person secretariat at NIMR. The secretariat coordinated quarterly meetings of the steering committee as well as cross-border regional meetings that included a larger collection of interested parties. The secretariat produced a monthly Web-based newsletter on regional disease data and a print circular (for rural locales where information technologies were less developed). The three countries agreed on a list of eighteen priority diseases for regional surveillance and moved toward standardized procedures in surveillance and response and a common format for reporting their activities. Other achievements included

---

59. L. E. G. Mboera et al., *Technical Report: East African Integrated Disease Surveillance Network, 2001–2004* (Dar es Salaam: National Institute for Medical Research, November 2004).
60. Ibid., 6.
61. Personal interview, Dar es Salaam, Tanzania, December 18, 2009; personal interview, New York, NY, December 22, 2009.

conducting a joint workshop on the use of computerized geographic information systems to improve disease tracking and identify weaknesses in response capabilities; sharing diagnostic skills and tools and standardization of public health curricula; and coordinating on a regional basis with global initiatives such as the GOARN and ProMED.[62]

Despite progress on several fronts, EAIDSNet did not develop into a robust regional cooperation network like MBDS and MECIDS. It was not able to elicit the full cooperation of the national ministries of health with regard to data sharing, a shortcoming that members attributed to several factors. First, the divergent national bureaucratic protocols for information control and sharing among member states inhibited cooperation. For example, an EAIDSNet's self-report laments the inability of border districts in two member countries from sharing urgent information about outbreaks with their regional neighbors:

> If a District Medical Officer sees an outbreak that could spread, he first has to send this information to his Ministry of Health, who passes it to the Ministry of Health in the neighboring country, who passes it down to the District Medical Officer at the border district on the other side of the border. This process is time consuming and often breaks down, and consequently information never reaches the border district.[63]

A second barrier to cooperation was the frequent turnover of key network participants, several of whom left their respective health ministries to accept other national appointments or to join international governmental bodies and, in one instance, to untimely death. The replacement of principals limited the degree of familiarity and confidence among the network's leadership. Finally, parallel initiatives on IDSR underway in the Great Lakes Region in East Africa led by the WHO's African Regional Office (WHO-AFRO) placed their own demands on national health ministries for surveillance and reporting improvements and drew resources away from the development of the sort of self-guided transgovernmental cooperation that was established in MBDS, which was the model for EAIDSNet.

Together these institutional, personnel, and procedural barriers reduced the effectiveness of EAIDSNet and impeded the creation of a trusted network of closely linked individuals that formed the foundation for sustained transnational surveillance and response in the Mekong and Middle East. EAIDSNet was not able to develop a regional infectious disease database from a common regional approach to disease reporting, nor did it make

---

62. Mboera et al., *Technical Report;* personal interview, Washington, DC, November 25, 2009.
63. Mboera et al., *Technical Report*, 44.

significant progress toward coordinated response to regional infectious disease outbreaks.

By 2004, EAIDSNet also faced the problem of securing additional financial and institutional resources to sustain its efforts at regional cooperation in infectious disease control. In its first three years, the Rockefeller Foundation was the only significant contributor to the EAIDSNet regional initiative. In 2004, the member state participants, the Rockefeller Foundation, and the EAC agreed to fold EAIDSNet into the Health Sub-Sector of the EAC Social Sector. The hand-off to the EAC was fully consistent with the community's treaty language, and it was hoped that a more official, intergovernmental organization like the EAC could remove bureaucratic barriers to information flows and secure greater commitment from the participants through its established institutions, committees, funding, and staff. With a second, three-year commitment of Rockefeller funds of $406,760 to hire a new health sector director and to relocate the secretariat to the EAC headquarters in Arusha, participants believed that EAIDS-Net's would be better able to sustain its activities because the EAC would eventually absorb the costs associated with strengthening infectious disease control as part of its social sector budget. The parties anticipated that during this second phase the network would strengthen communication and collaboration among the three original East African partner states in all aspects of disease surveillance, improve capacity in disease surveillance and control, and develop training programs for staff to implement disease surveillance and control activities.[64]

Although the strategy for the relocation of EAIDSNet to the EAC was sensible and perhaps necessary, it created an institutional hiatus and an absence of direct responsibility for network functions. In July 2005, the EAC convened the inaugural meeting of the Sub-Sectoral Council of Ministers of Health. At that and subsequent meetings, efforts to improve infectious disease control in the region became part of a larger public health agenda of a more formal, intergovernmental institution. Under the EAC, in addition to efforts to strengthen infectious disease surveillance, reporting, and response, the Health Sub-Sector also launched initiatives on community health and on integrating health-related research in the region. These programs speak to a wider range of public health challenges facing the region, are in varying states of progress, and have attracted external support in some instances. The cross-border network, however, has atrophied. EAC decisions are made through committees and established intergovernmental channels, in

---

64. East African Community, October 7, 2009. See also Mboera et al., *Technical Report*, 45–46.

contrast to the more formal, consensual network that was the operational mode for EAIDSNet.

CHORDS: Connecting Health Organizations for Regional Disease Surveillance

Representatives from MECIDS, MDBS, EAIDSNet, and other infectious disease surveillance networks from around the globe met together for the first time in December 2007 in Bellagio, Italy. The Global Health and Security Initiative gathered the experts to share best practices and lessons learned and to recommend the necessary actions to advance the global capacity for public health surveillance, with particular attention to infectious disease surveillance in developing countries.[65] Although MECIDS, MDBS, and EAIDSNet all focus on regional infectious disease surveillance and response, the international-level meeting was a response to a call to extend this cooperation to a global level.

In January 2008, building on the momentum created in Bellagio, many of the same infectious disease experts and other global leaders in public health launched a call for action to urge governments, international intergovernmental organizations, and private foundations to implement and carry forward a series of actions. In particular, the call to action committed the participants and called on others to

- strengthen national capacity and regional networks based on effective electronic communication, by regular meetings and joint projects;
- promote and enhance the overall global capacity for infectious disease surveillance by coordinating regional networks into a global cooperative activity;
- develop and encourage collaboration between the human, animal, and agricultural sectors to achieve a holistic approach to infectious disease surveillance; and
- promote development of national capacities and new regional networks, particularly in Africa and South Asia.

In response to this call for action, a new transnational NGO has emerged—Connecting Health Organizations for Regional Disease Surveillance. Representatives of MBDS, MECIDS, EAIDSNet and many other infectious disease surveillance and control experts gathered again in

---

65. Global Health and Security Initiative, "Projects: Connecting and Enhancing Regional Disease Surveillance Networks Around the World," www.ghsi.org/spotlight.html.

Washington, DC, in April 2009 to announce the launching of CHORDS and to discuss expanding it. Although CHORDS is being developed through GHSI, the initiative is being funded by $20 million from the Rockefeller Foundation through its Disease Surveillance Network Initiative to strengthen and further connect regional disease surveillance networks. Katherine Bond, the former associate director of the Rockefeller Foundation's Africa Regional Office in Nairobi Kenya, emphasized the need for the development of this network of disease surveillance networks, calling the networks a "new form of global health diplomacy" that has proved a "flexible and responsive means to work with, through and around more static institutional structures." The regional networks that have evolved with the assistance of funding from the Rockefeller Foundation are "serving as a common platform through which to coordinate efforts of multiple donors and other institutional partners and support the work of the World Health Organization and other bilateral and multilateral agencies by creating better coordination regionally and bilaterally and by participating in the Global Outbreak Alert and Response Network. Dr. Bond also reiterated that regional networks will, through the organizational capabilities of CHORDS, be able to "strengthen their own networks, share lessons across regions, and enhance global monitoring and reporting efforts."[66]

GHSI established working groups to develop strategies and materials for the second annual CHORDS Conference, which was held in March 2010 in Annecy, France. Ultimately, CHORDS aims to create a multifaceted community of practitioners and organizations to improve early detection and response in the regional networks and strengthen partnerships for global health security. The Rockefeller Foundation provided GHSI a grant for CHORDS to establish the steering committee, hire staff, and convene the 2010 CHORDS conference. With guidance from an international steering committee, CHORDS is striving to become a "community of practice" for disease surveillance and e-health experts to

- share standards and distribute common knowledge;
- harness the experience of disease surveillance experts in the animal, human, and agricultural sectors from around the world by collaborating on direct, interactive problem-solving;
- drive connectivity and improve knowledge management using a hybrid system of advanced tools and technologies;

---

66. Katherine Bond, "Promoting Trans-National Collaboration in Disease Surveillance and Control" (presentation, The Rockefeller Foundation Africa Regional Office, Nairobi, Kenya, April 28, 2009), www.rockfound.org/about_us/speeches/042809swine_flu_k_bond.shtml.

- help participating countries meet their legal obligations under the 2005 International Health Regulations; and
- make recommendations and generate support to sustain and develop regional disease surveillance networks.[67]

CHORDS is the first systematic attempt to coordinate higher-level political integration among the regional infectious disease networks. Although new, it is a development that warrants attention to determine if it is a sustainable form of neofunctional institutional growth.

Conclusion

This chapter has outlined the progress of the three transnational initiatives in infectious disease control. These networks operate at a mezzanine level between global and pan-regional architectures and national public health systems, and are part of an important emerging example of interstate cooperation and transnational governance—issues that are the foci of the next two chapters.

---

67. Global Health and Security Initiative, "Projects: Connecting Health Organizations for Regional Disease Surveillance (CHORDS)," www.ghsi.org/projects/chords.html.

3

THE THREE '*I*'S OF INTERNATIONAL COOPERATION: INTEREST, INSTITUTIONS, AND IDENTITY

With regard to international cooperation, the three cases present a paradox. The states of the Mekong Basin could not be more varied in their governance structures and levels of economic attainment. Throughout the Cold War era and since, these countries have known frequent intraregional conflict. Yet, under MBDS, they cooperate closely and continuously on a matter of great sensitivity to national security and welfare. Likewise, MECIDS began during the Second Intifada and sustained itself during a period of rising political tensions and violence, including the hostilities in Gaza. In East Africa, several of the participants have struggled with internal violence, severe economic constraints, and an uneven history of regional cooperation and estrangement, and yet managed to launch a complex cooperative initiative. This chapter offers a preliminary explanation for this anomalous cooperation occurring among traditional adversaries and in troubled or resource poor environments. The explanation for cooperation lies in three, interrelated processes: securing shared interests in an important transnational public good; creating and maintaining institutional arrangements that are appropriately inclusive, practical, equitable, and efficacious; and redefining identities so as to include formerly excluded actors in one's salient in-group affiliation and developing trust among members of the new inclusive group.

Why Cooperation: Securing Common Interests in a Transnational Public Good

Absent the prospect for meaningful new gains, states and their private and public collaborators have limited motivation to overcome the challenges to cooperation. States participate in transnational initiatives to obtain interests they could not otherwise secure, and it is the overlapping of interests among states and nonstate actors that can be seen as the central or necessary condition for transnational cooperative efforts.[1] A transnational initiative must have the potential to create a collaborative advantage, that is, some significant welfare enhancing benefit that could not be achieved without the collaboration. Furthermore, the value created must flow to all core members.[2]

Preventing and controlling infectious disease outbreak and the health benefits related to doing so are a shared interest in a public good best secured regionally or transnationally. In general, securing public goods is difficult and capturing the benefits of transnational public goods even more problematic. Public goods are those that yield benefits that are nonrival in consumption (can be enjoyed simultaneously by all in a specific community) and nonexcludable (from which no one in the community can be kept from consuming).[3] At a local level, for example, a public good could be the enjoyment of a city park, or at a national level, the sense of security from foreign invasion provided to all citizens by the existence of a national army or militia.

The paradox of public goods, of course, is that they tend to be underprovided. Because they are nonexcludable, a price cannot be enforced and thus no private incentive exists to produce them.[4] The paradox can be overcome at the local and national level to the extent that the government can enforce production, such as by taxing citizens for the provision of a city park or by conscripting soldiers for an army.

For global and regional transnational public goods, however, the problem is more difficult because (as realists rightly underscore) no global or regional government finances and enforces public goods production. Absent a formal government with such powers, the multilateral actors involved in providing a regional or global public good must rely on recognizing their enlightened self-interest. Enlightened self-interest is composed of self-interest, shared

---

1.   Marco Schaferhoff, Sabine Campe, and Christopher Kaan, "Transnational Public-Private Partnerships in International Relations: Making Sense of Concepts, Research Frameworks, and Results," *International Studies Review* 11, no. 3 (2009): 456–57.

2.   Chris Huxham and Siv Vangen, "What Makes Partnerships Work?" in *Public-Private Partnerships: Theory and Practice in International Perspective*, ed. Stephen P. Osborne, 293–310 (London: Routledge, 2000); Michael R. Reich, "Introduction: Public-Private Partnerships for Public Health," in *Public-Private Partnerships for Public Health*, 1–18 (Cambridge, MA: Harvard Series on Population and International Health, Harvard Center for Population and Development Studies, April 2002).

3.   Richard Smith et al., "Communicable Disease Control: A Global Public Good Perspective," *Health Policy and Planning* 15, no. 5 (2004): 271–78; Scott Barrett, *Why Cooperate? The Incentive to Supply Global Public Goods* (New York: Oxford University Press, 2007).

4.   The European Union is a possible exception to this generalization.

interest, and altruism (other-interest) that together enhance one's well-being.[5] As all theoretical perspectives can agree, recognizing and acting collectively on one's enlightened self-interest is rare in international relations; it does not happen just because one believes it should happen from an ethical or logical standpoint. Cooperation is particularly vexatious when it touches on the security of the state and the states in question, as here, have little or no history of cooperation.

Why are MBDS, MECIDS, and, for a time, EAIDSNet, exceptional in their ability to overcome the barriers to the production of a sensitive transnational public good, especially when the organizations' membership includes countries without a strong history of cooperation? I suggest three reasons. First, it is in the clear self-interest of each member to control transboundary communicable diseases. As noted in chapter 1, it is increasingly the responsibility of states to provide for the health of their populations. Second, infectious disease control is a public good that creates a consumption externality, that is, preventing or treating an infectious disease not only benefits the patient, but also benefits others by reducing their risk of infection. Likewise, the control of a communicable disease in a given country reduces the likelihood of an outbreak in an adjacent country if the two countries share common food, air, and water or other vectors of interdependence. If each country receives substantial consumption externalities from another's control of infectious disease, then both are more likely to appreciate and act on their shared interest in disease control.[6] Furthermore, because of their physical interdependence, the mutual benefit arising from infectious disease control is readily apparent and the consequences of failing to cooperate are equally clear to all. In this sense, vulnerability to infectious disease outbreak and spread is a classic and compelling superordinate problem because infectious disease affects each member, is shared by all, and cannot be resolved without joint action. As one author suggests, "the vicious threat posed by diseases and pathogenic microbes . . . is predicated on . . . the mutuality of vulnerability."[7] Because of their proximity, network participants are keenly

---

5.   John E. Ikerd, "Rethinking the Economics of Self-Interest" (conference paper presented at the Organization for Comparative Markets, Omaha, NE, September 1999); Colin J. McInnes, "Looking Beyond the National Interest: Restructuring the Debate on Health and Foreign Policy," *Medical Journal of Australia* 180 (2004): 168–70.

6.   Depending on the biological properties of the disease and other environmental factors, the control of certain communicable diseases (for example, malaria) may be a transnational regional public good, while the control of other diseases (such as influenza) may constitute both a regional and a global public good.

7.   Obijiofor Aginam, *Global Health Governance: International Law and Public Health in a Divided World* (Toronto: University of Toronto Press, 2005), 3.

and directly aware of their mutual vulnerability and that national efforts alone will not protect their populations. Third, their shared vulnerability both underscores the benefits of securing mutual interests and infuses an element of altruism into state calculations. Public health officials, by virtue of their training and current responsibilities, are particularly sensitive to the indivisible nature of their shared vulnerability. MBDS actors, for example, expressed empathetic understanding of the problem their cohorts in other member states faced and showed no interest in blaming each other for past outbreaks. They stressed that the dangers in this area of public health are serious, and, as scientists, recognized that infectious disease could arise in any part of the region at any time.[8]

Taken together, states can more readily appreciate and act on their enlightened self-interest in providing a regional public good when interdependence (both positive and negative) is acute and where positive externalities exist. Recent pandemic scares such as SARS and avian flu added a sense of urgency to national efforts. With regard to infectious disease control, the six countries of the MBDS system, the three political entities of MECIDS, and the three founding countries of the EAIDSNet each faced a problem with a clear and compelling win-win-win-win solution, not just win-win: by cooperating on infectious disease control, I benefit, you benefit, I benefit by you benefiting, and vice versa. As one MECIDS principal explained, in infectious disease protection, "You are only as strong as your neighbor."[9] Also, each actor can take credit for any successful results from cooperation because this benefit is also nonrival and nonexclusive. This latter feature helps to ensure political support from participating countries' health ministers.

Why Cooperation: Institutional Arrangements

It is not only the compelling public good of infectious disease control and the vivid superordinate problem of infectious disease outbreak that ensure cooperation. Many international public goods and superordinate, transnational regional and global problems are awaiting effective transnational action, such as the protection or sustainable use of important aspects of the natural environment, the containment of terrorism, and the prevention of transnational human rights violations. Rather, it is the combination of this compelling benefit and the particular fit between the agent (MBDS or MECIDS in particular) and the action (transnational infectious disease

---

8.   Personal interview, Bangkok, Thailand, April 6–10, 2009.
9.   Personal interview, Swaimeh, Jordan, October 31, 2009.

control) that is critical to success. Here is where institutional arrangements become important to explaining cooperation, as liberals emphasize.

Specifically, the size and composition of MBDS and MECIDS memberships facilitate effective cooperation in disease surveillance and response where other groupings fall short. In many, perhaps most, international configurations, the provision of global public goods remains inchoate or merely an aspiration in part because the members do not share enough benefits or are not so interdependent as to fully appreciate and act on the existence of shared interests or vulnerabilities.

The cases of MBDS and MECIDS best illustrate this point. The Mekong Basin Disease Surveillance network is composed of six bordering countries whose water, air, and food regularly transgress political boundaries. Because of physical proximity and growing commercial relations among some of the countries, the Mekong Basin is an increasingly interdependent region. MBDS membership includes all the relevant parties and none that are irrelevant in addressing the problem of infectious disease spread in this Asian subregion. Compare MBDS membership with the Southeast Asian Region of the WHO. As noted, in 1948 WHO assumed responsibility over existing international sanitary regulations from its predecessor under the League of Nations and organized itself into six regional offices.[10] For particular political and historical reasons, its Southeast Asian region includes eleven countries ranging from the Democratic People's Republic of Korea (North Korea), to India, to Thailand, to Timor-Leste, but does not include Laos, Cambodia, southern China, or Vietnam. Thailand, as a member of the Southeast Asian region, has little to no common interest in or ability to conduct disease surveillance and response with North Korea under the WHO structure, but every reason to want to work closely with Laos, Cambodia, southern China, and Vietnam in MBDS. Likewise, in the case of MECIDS, eighty miles separate the capitals of the three political entities. Under existing international arrangements, however, Jordan and the Palestinian Authority fall under the jurisdiction of the WHO's Eastern Mediterranean region. Israel, which sits cheek-by-jowl with these two nations, is part of the WHO's European region, thus complicating already difficult conditions for joint action. Simply put, the right institutional membership is critical to securing a shared public good and solving a superordinate problem—even one as critical as infectious disease control. As Renate Mayntz explains, effective collaborative problem solving depends on a congruence between the causal

---

10. As noted, the six regions are Africa, Southeast Asia, the Americas, the eastern Mediterranean, Europe, and the western Pacific.

agents (those who produce the problem) and the potential problem solvers (those actors capable of effecting a solution).[11]

The right players are needed in other senses too, for example, the network decision makers must have the authority to speak for their respective health ministries and, indirectly, their governments. Absent actors able to get things done back home, these networks would be essentially powerless. In two of the three networks, powerful state actors in the form of the leading public health officials were essential to the network's success. A host of other institutional and procedural factors facilitate successful cooperation, which I address in the next chapter, in a detailed discussion of what constitutes effective transnational governance.

Why Cooperation: Redefining Identity and Interests

As the constructivist perspective rightly notes, the identity of actors and their concomitant interests are not fully fixed in international relations. It is necessary, when examining the issue of cooperation, to consider how interaction shapes and reshapes these two critical factors. In two of these three cases, there is much more than a confluence of interest among relevant actors: there is also the steady construction by political elites and professionals of what Bruce Cronin calls a "transnational political community," a group that shares a common identity across political boundaries.[12] A transnational political community can develop when "a set of political actors sharing a common social characteristic, a common relationship, a common experience, and a positive interdependence develop a political consciousness that defines them as a unique group."[13] Not only does it secure common goods, a community also shares a sense of self and its members have a stake in maintaining positive internal relations in the group (call it an interest in securing the common good rather than the common goods). Creating a community ensures that the cooperation achieved by the group, as in the cases of MBDS and MECIDS, is not ad hoc or opportunistic.

These groups derive their meaning from the interaction of the political actors, which is evident in their discourse and patterns of behavior, which

---

11. Renate Mayntz, "From Government to Governance: Political Steering in Modern Societies" (paper presented at the Summer Academy of International Public Policy, Wuerzburg, September 7–11, 2003), 7–8.

12. Bruce Cronin, *Community under Anarchy: Transnational Identity and the Evolution of Cooperation* (New York: Columbia University Press, 1999), 3. A common transnational identity means members of a group categorize themselves as sharing behavioral and personal or corporate characteristics with actors outside their juridical borders.

13. Ibid., 4.

both reflect a shared sense of self. It is difficult to quantify this variable and, though one could count up the interactions across nodes in the network,[14] it is more important to assess the quality of those interactions. How do the actors characterize each other, do they acknowledge the group and indicate their desire to be part of it? The quality of group behavior and interactions is also important evidence of a shift in identity. Do these actors pursue shared interests consistent with a common identity? Does their action reflect group cohesion, consensus, and solidarity?

The evidence from the cases illustrate that MBDS and MECIDS have created an effective transnational problem-solving network with a strong, shared identity among members, whereas EAIDSNet did not. MBDS, for example, grew out of the response of health professionals to an unmet need: detecting and responding to transboundary infectious disease. The organization's founders all had an abiding professional commitment to the public health of their populations and were not just nominally committed to the problem or in a great hurry to have a political success to show for their efforts. The key actors describe themselves as working people, and not as political figures or even policymakers, even though they are political officials and keenly aware of their highly charged regional politics. Over time, MBDS leaders became quite familiar with each other through their regular interactions within MBDS and other international public health forums.

Similarly, in MECIDS, initial suspicions of the other were quickly overcome by the scientific and practical values and professional similarities shared by the participants, characteristics underscored by the conveners and NGO facilitators. Carefully constructed initial encounters and repeated interactions leading to tangible progress and goal achievement reinforced the membership's common identity despite the lack of a formal institutional status.

In contrast, divergent levels of interest in the network, frequent turnover of key personnel, and competing institutional loyalties limited the ability of EAIDSNet to forge an enduring network of trust. For this reason, among others, EAIDSNet, of necessity, merged into a larger, more formal, transnational institution with a broader public health mandate.

How do we account for the creation of a transnational identity or transnational community in theoretical terms? If national identity dominates in world politics and this identity and its corresponding interests are relatively fixed, then when and how can traditionally weak transnational identities be created, strengthened, and engaged to solve regional or global problems?

---

14. Emilie M. Hafner-Burton, Miles Kahler, and Alexander H. Montgomery, "Networked Analysis for International Relations," *International Organization* 63 (Summer 2009): 559–92.

How is a transnational identity shaped from a collection of ostensibly national actors? International relations theory offers limited guidance on this point.[15] Instead, social psychology offers a more explicit theoretical account of how a group identity forms through social interactions among selves, whether individual or corporate.

Specifically, social identity theory (SIT) can help us understand the difficult process of altering group identification. SIT experiments have repeatedly demonstrated that to make their cognitive environment manageable, individuals and groups organize their understanding of the social world on the basis of categorical distinctions and comparisons between their in-group (self) and the out-group (other).[16] Once categorization and comparison occur, demonstrable cognitive, emotional, and behavioral consequences follow. Specifically, categorization leads to the tendency to accentuate in-group sameness and out-group differences,[17] generate positive affect (trust and liking) of the in-group and suspicion of the out-group, and behavior that rewards disproportionately the members of the in-group and punishes disproportionately the members of the out-group.[18] SIT illustrates the very real challenge of constructing mutually beneficial relations once a distinction between in-group and out-group is in place, such as national identities. In this sense, social identity can reinforce the barriers to cooperation noted by political realists.[19]

SIT also explains how these categories can change through social interactions, as constructivists suggest, and how new social groupings and interests are formed through recategorization and redefinition of self. Because actors' identities are socially constructed by the conceptual distinctions they em-

---

15. A notable exception is William Bloom, *Personal Identity, National Identity, and International Relations* (Cambridge: Cambridge University Press, 1990). Bloom is primarily interested in the question of how individuals develop a shared sense of nationhood through a process he calls identification. With regard to moving beyond national identity toward transnational identity, Bloom believes that this expansion of identity is possible when there is a clear symbolic form with which identification takes place (the European Union, for example); that form evokes identification by being protective in the face of external threat, and the new group identification is seen as materially beneficial.

16. See Marilynn B. Brewer, "When Contact Is Not Enough: Social Identity and Intergroup Cooperation," *International Journal of Intercultural Relations* 20, nos. 3/4 (1996): 291–303, citing the research of Henri Tajfel and John C. Turner, "The Social Identity Theory of Intergroup Behavior," in *Psychology of Intergroup Relations*, eds. Stephen Worchel and William Austin (Chicago: Nelson Hall, 1986) 7–24.

17. Competition is the natural response to the perception of negative interdependence.

18. See Henri Tajfel, "Experiments in Intergroup Discrimination," *Scientific American* 223, no. 5 (November 1970): 96–102.

19. Jonathan Mercer relies on SIT to argue for the inherent competition built into international relations based on cognitions and categorizations that are prior to interactions, in distinction to constructivists' claims that, prior to interaction, international relations are neither competitive nor cooperative. "Anarchy and Identity," *International Organization* 49, no. 2 (Spring 1995): 229–52.

brace, identity and interests are recognized as potentially malleable and that the self has multiple, overlapping identities manifesting in different ways in different contexts. This is not to say that a transnational identity develops easily or that systemic anarchy and sovereignty do not constrain its evolution. They do, but sovereignty is not an impenetrable barrier everywhere to transnational community building.[20] Even in anarchy, social interaction can transform identity or alter the salience of particular identity. It can redefine who is in the in-group, who is outside this conceptual boundary, and which identity takes priority in a particular setting.[21]

SIT holds that a transformation of identity can occur when actors develop attachment to selective others through recategorization, recomparison, and re-identification. The process requires contact, perception of some shared characteristics among members, a shared exclusive relationship, and a high level of shared interest and potential for mutual reward, ideally in an area of primary need.[22] As the new group is defined to include previously foreign actors and conceptual separations are diminished, trust is promoted, and collective action problems become more tractable.

Contact is a necessary starting point. The contact hypothesis supports the conclusion that a necessary (but not sufficient) condition for the reduction of intergroup conflict and prejudice is some form of cooperative interdependence in pursuit of common superordinate goals. Decategorization through personalization is based on the idea that contact will be most effective if interactions are highly personal rather than categorical.[23] Interaction at this level reduces depersonalization that is the consequence of prior categorization. Individual interactions reduce the salience of categorical distinctions, negative stereotypes, and the tendency to discount the possibility of positive interdependence that is typical of in-group bias.[24] Meaningful and real experience of the other can trigger a new process of categorization.

The early meetings of the three networks illustrate this decategorizing through personalizing and recategorizing in promoting a new, more inclusive group. The networks' meetings were carefully orchestrated by

---

20. Cronin, *Community under Anarchy*, 21. William Bloom captures this point artfully: "Philosophically, identification may be a selfish drive—and, practically, it may be conducted aggressively and sometimes fatally—but socially it is by its nature cooperative and adaptive." *Personal Identity*, 45.

21. Cronin, *Community under Anarchy*, 17. Mercer, who relies on SIT theory to account for the underlying competitive nature of international relations, nonetheless acknowledges that one's in group can be altered and expanded. He cites the creation of the European Union as an example. "Anarchy and Identity," 250, 252.

22. Cronin, *Community under Anarchy*, 31.

23. Brewer, "When Contact Is Not Enough," 293.

24. Ibid.

participating NGOs precisely to emphasize the personally and professionally shared characteristics of the participants as scientists and public health professionals facing a common threat. Superordinate goals—in these cases the reduction of infectious disease outbreaks in vulnerable populations—were used as part of social interaction to reduce intergroup hostility and to make more salient a new unitary group. In addition, common culture characteristics abetted cooperation in some of the networks.[25]

If successful, the process is marked by a cognitive and affective shift, in terms of loyalty and trust, to encompass the new, larger team. With the perception of a new single entity rather than the mere aggregation of two separate groups comes a more positive attitude and approach to formerly out-group members.

Evidence from two of the cases is particularly striking on this point. The merger of formerly separate, often antagonistic, identities is reflected in the memberships' characterization of the new group. MECIDS principals often refer to the group as like family and to their counterparts as friends or brothers, a discourse also used by MBDS members.[26] Soon after the organization was formed, MECIDS principals began to recognize each other as common health professionals. This shared profession is the locus for two common characteristics they repeatedly cite as bases for understanding and institutional success. First, as scientists and physicians, they share a common language with relatively precise and undifferentiated meanings, unlike diplomats, who are practiced in the art of finding mutually agreeable words designed to accommodate multiple interpretations. As one MECIDS official put it, "Morbidity is morbidity, a reagent is a reagent, . . . I know what he [his MECIDS counterpart] is thinking."[27] Second, as public health physicians, they share certain common values such as a perceived duty of care, especially for the poorest and least fortunate members of their respective populations.

Decategorizing and recategorizing require practice: protracted and positive contact that allows perceptions of common characteristics and shared interests to be identified and reinforced. Discreet but regular interactions among members of the two most successful networks is a distinguishing characteristic of their practice. The founding efforts of each organization reflect the advice of Chris Huxam and Siv Vangan: "If you are seriously

---

25. The literature on international relations and cooperation has looked at culture to explain elements of state and interstate behavior. See Peter Katzenstein, ed., *The Culture of National Security* (Princeton, NJ: Princeton University Press, 1996).

26. Personal interview, Bangkok, Thailand, April 6–10, 2009; personal interview, Swaimeh, Jordan, October 30–31, 2009.

27. Personal interview, Swaimeh, Jordan, October 31, 2009.

concerned to achieve success in [a public-private governance] partnership, be prepared to nurture . . . and nurture . . . and nurture."[28]

Positive interdependence also contributed to group reclassification in the cases of MBDS and MECIDS. Their members actively and successfully engaged in real world problem-solving activities that they came to view as significant positive achievements. As one MECIDS member said, "If this [organization] was just talk, I would not come to the meetings."[29] MBDS and MECIDS are practice communities, not just knowledge (epistemic) communities and not just "talk-shops," though, as noted, principals share professions and scientific understandings, and communicate regularly both at formal meetings and informally. MBDS and MECIDS interactions are grounded in common and continuous practice in disease surveillance, detection, and response. Members from all three networks recognize the creation of mutual benefits in an area of essential need as the result of their creation of a new entity.

Although tangible steps marked the progress of the two most successful groups, their efforts were not subjected to strict, politically determined timetables. MBDS and MECIDS evolved over time. The MBDS network began a decade ago without significant political fanfare or scrutiny. At the onset, it was an informal gathering focused on training exercises, identifying lessons learned, and building capacity among public health physicians and scientists. For example, in the case of MBDS, the impetus for the organizations came from an INGO working with senior health officials from Cambodia, Laos, and Thailand (by virtue of geographic centrality) who drew from earlier bilateral exchanges on matters of public health. Three years into its operation, the health ministers of the six countries signed a two-page MOU, giving MBDS a quasi-official status. Foreign ministries or heads of state never formally endorsed MBDS at a higher level. Technically speaking, MBDS is not a legal entity and has only a modest budget that does not come directly from any of the member states. This structure allows for flexibility of operation and less political posturing or undue interference. The organizational history allowed a network of trusted relationships to grow organically over time and without unrealistic expectations or artificial timetables. The organization did not develop by fiat, but rather from an unmet need, and it grew by members working together in identifying and responding to difficult and sensitive problems. It evolved from the ground up, not from the top down. The key actors were free to define and act on the problems they identified

---

28. Huxham and Vangan, "What Makes Partnerships Work?" 307.
29. Personal interview, Swaimeh, Jordan, October 31, 2009.

on site—not problems identified by donors or a remote international bureaucracy. By working together on the problems they believed were critical, the organization developed a sense of efficacy, and its members developed familiarity and trust. As MBDS evolved, membership expanded slightly (adding a second Chinese provincial government), and the agenda grew as new infectious disease challenges emerged and to keep pace with the official goals of IHR 2005. The MBDS institutional structure has gradually become more extensive to better manage its expanding workload. As its agenda expands and MBDS enters a new phase of its cooperation, questions arise as to whether the personal relationships so critical to its early success can be replicated and institutionalized.

MECIDS has followed a similar pattern of steady trust and institution building. Repeated interaction and problem solving for more than six years has built lines of communication across national boundaries and trust among the leadership of MECIDS. They know both whom to call, and that they can rely on what they are told. The actors take pride in the organization's growing capacity, they view its accomplishments as significant, and they see tangible benefits flowing from their affiliation with the organization. EAIDSNet, in its initial years also developed some of these ties, but it was unable to sustain its network of relationships.

When decategorization and recategorization begin to take hold, the emergence of trust and the securing of collective goods become possible. Trust is the essential norm of these transnational disease surveillance groups.[30] Trust was built over time from regular group interaction, the reliability of the information shared among the members of a group, and joint problem solving. Many MBDS professionals, for example, have worked together in the organization for seven or eight years and are in regular electronic communication. They also interact as representatives of their countries at more formal regional and global conclaves. MBDS and MECIDS officials are consciously attempting to perpetuate a sense of friendship, kinship, and organizational commitment through training exercises and other meetings that engage the next generation of health officials.

A word on trust is in order to appreciate fully its importance in supporting and sustaining cooperation, because the concept of trust not only helps us understand how cooperation is possible, it also helps explain how behavioral practices evolve from the interaction of a small group of individuals

---

30. On the importance of trust in public-private partnerships see Erik-Hans Klijn and Geert R. Teisman, "Governing Public-Private Partnerships," in *Public–Private Partnerships: Theory and Practice in International Perspective*, ed. Stephen P. Osborne, (London: Routledge, 2000) 84–102.

to a larger (transnational) system. Understanding trust, like understanding identity, also requires a sociological detour because international relations theory typically reduces trust to its calculative component and fails to appreciate its full significance in explaining cooperation.[31] Trust is more than just a calculation, it is a social phenomenon contingent on interpersonal relations and circumstances. Individuals would have no occasion to trust or need to trust apart from social relationships. Trust also is a property of collective units (dyads, groups, organizations, and large collectivities).

Trust, although a multifaceted and contested term, can be defined as a "belief that others will not deliberately or knowingly do us harm, if they can avoid it, and will look after our interests, if this is possible."[32] Trust has three key underlying conditions: a degree of interdependence among actors, an element of risk or uncertainty in exchange relationships, and an expectation that the vulnerability resulting from the acceptance of risk will not be taken advantage of by the other party in the relationship. When these bases are in place, trust is seen behaviorally as the undertaking of a course of action that involves some risk in the confident expectation that others involved in the interaction will act as expected and desired. Trust is indispensable in social relationships, which, because of imperfect information, always involve an unavoidable element of risk.[33]

Trust can bridge the micro (interpersonal) level and the macro (systemic) level of analysis. The micro level is typically interpersonal trust between individuals based on familiarity developed in previous direct interaction or derived from membership in the same social group. Typically, trust is built in a series of small steps. Larger entities, in turn, are seen as trustworthy to the extent they have developed a culture, which, although it originated in the interaction of critical individuals, now has been institutionalized in

31. See, for example, Andrew H. Kydd, *Trust and Mistrust in International Relations* (Princeton, NJ: Princeton University Press, 2005). Trust has two broad bases: a calculative/cognitive base and an emotional/normative base that are comingled in varying measures in any particular social experience. Calculative trust involves expectations about another, based on evidence-based reasoning, which weighs the costs and benefits of certain courses of action to an actor seeking to maximize his or her utility. Social trust is also constructed on an emotional base that complements its calculative dimension. This affective component is an emotional bond among those who participate in the relationship. The sharing of common values among individuals is indispensable to the formation of this aspect of trust. Talcott Parsons and others see trust as emerging from a relationship that, through repeated interactions and processes, creates a consensus in values and norms of obligation or "solidarity." *The Social System* (London: Routledge & Kegan Paul, 1951). See also Christel Lane, "Introduction: Theories and Issues in the Study of Trust," in *Trust Within and Between Organizations*, eds. Christel Lane and Reinhard Bachmann (Oxford: Oxford University Press, 1998), 1–30.

32. Kenneth Newton, "Social and Political Trust," in *The Oxford Handbook of Political Behavior*, eds. Russell J. Dalton and Hans-Dieter Klingemann, (Oxford: Oxford University Press, 2007), 343–44.

33. J. David Lewis and Andrew Weigert, "Trust as a Social Concept," *Social Forces* 63, no. 4 (June 1985): 968, citing Georg Simmel, *The Philosophy of Money* (London: Routledge & Kegan Paul, 1978).

decision-making mechanisms and systems that reward trusting behavior. So-called boundary-spanning persons can shorten the process of building trust in exchange relationships through their regular personal contacts thereby moving trust from characteristic- or process-based trust to institutional-based trust.[34] System trust is built up by ongoing affirmative experiences associated with using the system. At present, the MBDS and MECIDS networks are young organizations transitioning from the highly personalized trust associated with small groups to more institutionalized trust that rests equally on the reliable performance of established procedures and favorable outcomes. Building this institutional trust is an ongoing process the principals recognize as necessary to sustainable success.

Trust takes time to establish and is not easy to sustain; its actual continuance in any particular social relationship is always problematic. Trust requires consistent effort. On the other hand, motives and rewards for making the effort to sustain a trusting relationship are clear. System trust improves efficiency; reduces transactions cost to initiating, monitoring, and enforcing agreements; and hence can be attractive to participants and self-reinforcing. Most organization scholars associate trust with highly positive effects on performance.[35] Concerns about damaging future gains from the trusted relationship or damaging one's reputation for trustworthiness also reinforce and help sustain trusted networks. Particularly important for disease surveillance cooperation, high levels of trust can lead to improved quantity, quality, and timeliness of information sharing among the partners and to the pooling of resources, and may highlight new avenues for cooperation.[36]

To summarize, creating a new inclusive group identification and a trusted network of cooperation is possible in international relations, but difficult and arduous. The steps that encourage decategorization and recategorization to include those previously characterized as other include contact, identifying and accentuating common characteristics, practicing problem solving and positive interdependence, and producing practical results that create value that rewards each participant's efforts. These steps can create a new, shared identity, engender trust, and enhance cooperation.

---

34. Jeffrey L. Bradach and Robert G. Eccles, "Price, Authority, and Trust: From Ideal Types to Plural Forms," *Annual Review of Sociology* 15, no. 1 (1989): 97–118.

35. Kenneth Arrow, *The Limits of Organization* (New York: W. W. Norton, 1974).

36. On the importance of political trust within societies, see Robert Putnam, *Making Democracy Work: Civic Tradition in Modern Italy* (Princeton, NJ: Princeton University Press, 1994); on trust in the private sector, see Mari Sako, *Prices, Quality and Trust: Inter-Firm Relations in Britain and Japan* (Cambridge: Cambridge University Press, 1992).

But can they "build a bridge to peace" and be the leading edge of wider cooperation through functional or neofunctional spillover into analogous functional or political issues? The cases recommend only a cautious enthusiasm. There is definite evidence that cooperation in the targeted issue area (infectious disease control) can deepen over time. In fact, expanding their mandates in infectious disease control is a consistent feature of both MBDS and MECIDS. Functional spillover into related issue areas, has been limited thus far. Time will tell. There are some early examples of functional cooperation in natural disaster planning and response and there are hopes for cooperation on issues such as bioterrorism. Neofunctional political collaboration is faint in the Mekong Basin and virtually absent in the case of Jordanian-Israeli-Palestinian relations. That MECIDS endures despite the lack of high-level diplomatic progress in the region is the silver lining in an otherwise dark landscape. Across regions, there is a nascent effort to combine these and other infectious disease initiatives into a larger network of networks under the CHORDS program and, as discussed in the next chapter, the networks generally work well with global initiatives under WHO.

Conclusion: Implications for International Cooperation Theory

This chapter offers a blended theory of international cooperation, that is, one that melds the variables of interest, institutions, and identity to account for largely unnoticed, but critical, examples of transnational cooperation. In the absence of central authority, cooperation in a sensitive matter related to national security and welfare depends on a compelling shared interest, convening and correctly engaging the right actors, and building a measure of shared identity and modicum of trust among individuals and within the new collaborative organization.

The practitioner community is correct in identifying many of the pieces of the puzzle: superordinate problems, shared interests, and common identity built around shared scientific and professional characteristics. This chapter illustrates how these pieces and others fit together into a coherent explanation for transnational cooperation in health.

International cooperation is not always possible, and, when available, can be painfully difficult to secure. The cases reveal that successful cooperation takes insight, imagination, risk-taking leaders, talented individuals, deft organizations, and lots of dedicated effort. Paraphrasing Max Weber, transnational cooperation in difficult regions "is the strong and slow boring of hard boards."[37] Nonetheless, international cooperation is possible and infectious disease control is not the only transnational problem amenable to cooperation between and among nations without a strong history of trust and amity. Other issue areas, such as counterterrorism cooperation, nuclear fuel regulation to discourage weapons proliferation, protection and allocation of critical natural resources (particularly water) at a regional and global level, prohibitions on human trafficking, and many more could benefit by the creation of trusted networks to secure public goods. Although each of these issues would present its own unique obstacles to cooperation and each set of actors their own set of antipathies to overcome, the sustained success of two of these three infectious disease control networks stand as a proof of concept that transnational cooperation is available in the practice of international relations in critical issues areas and among partners without a strong history of collaboration.

---

37. Peter Lassman and Ronald Speirs, eds., *Weber: Political Writings* (Cambridge: Cambridge University Press, 1994), 369.

4

PUBLIC-PRIVATE PARTNERSHIPS: TRANSNATIONAL GOVERNANCE IN REGIONAL DISEASE CONTROL

Transnational governance refers to those institutional arrangements beyond the nation-state in which private actors, usually as international nongovernmental organizations (INGOs) and transnational corporations (TNCs), participate in mixed public-private policy networks.[1] The purpose of these hybrid entities is to directly provide common goods and collectively solve problems by setting and implementing rules, and providing services.[2] This engagement with private actors should be distinguished analytically from the activities of private actors on the one hand in lobbying or attempting to influence states or international organizations (so-called networked advocacy), and on the other in directly providing services once the province of governments (so-called private governance).[3]

Transnational public-private governance also implies nonhierarchical steering, in contrast to hierarchic modes of governance, which characterize states or corporations acting alone. In transnational networks, states are active, even indispensable players, but are also embedded in a larger association involving complex and multidirectional interactions with nonstate actors in which responsibilities are shared and policies largely the product

---

1. Some scholars object to the word *partnership* as coloring the analysis of these organizations with a salutary term. Despite this concern, the term is widely used. For example, WHO describes partnership as a "means to bring together a set of actors for the common good of improving health of populations based on mutually agreed roles and principles." Ilona Kickbusch and Jonathan Quick, "Partnership for Health in the 21st Century," *World Health Statistics Quarterly* 51 (1998): 68–74.
2. Thomas Risse, "Transnational Governance and Legitimacy" (unpublished paper, Center for Transatlantic Foreign and Security Policy, Otto Suhr Institute of Political Science, Frie Universitat Berlin, February 2, 2004), 3–4; Renate Mayntz, "From Government to Governance: Political Steering in Modern Societies;" Rod A. W. Rhodes, *Understanding Governance: Policy Networks, Governance, Reflexivity, and Accountability* (Basingstoke: Macmillan, 1997).
3. Risse, "Transnational Governance," 3.

of negotiated consensus.[4] Compliance depends on the actor's perceptions of costs and benefits and the perceived 'legitimacy' of the rules and the rule-making process.[5]

Transnational public-private networks are organized around functional issues at various geographical levels and in varying configurations to address a host of governance problems in public health, biodiversity protection, climate change, economic regulation, humanitarian aid, security, and more. Some scholars see the emergence of transnational governance networks as constituting "a fundamental transformation in the organization of political authority in modern societies" or a "fundamental reconstitution of the global public domain."[6] Regardless of their ultimate significance, however, transnational public-private networks are undeniably more numerous and increasingly influential in raising and solving problems at a regional, and occasionally, at a global level.[7]

Such partnerships in health have expanded rapidly in the past two decades in various areas, including infectious disease control. They aim to produce and share international public goods,[8] and to go beyond traditional intergovernmental cooperation in health through the WHO or the World Bank to include industry and nongovernmental organizations in a new form of health governance.[9] Their names vary: global health

---

4.   Marie-Laurie Djelic and Kerstin Sahlin-Andersen, "Introduction: A World of Governance: The Rise of Transnational Regulation," in *Transnational Governance: Institutional Dynamics of Regulation*, eds. Marie-Laurie Djelic and Kerstin Sahlin-Andersen (Cambridge: Cambridge University Press, 2006), 1–28.

5.   Risse, "Transnational Governance and Legitimacy," 5. See also Ian Hurd, "Legitimacy and Authority in International Politics," *International Organization* 53, no. 2 (1999): 387.

6.   Edgar Grande and Louis W. Pauly, "Reconstituting Political Authority: Sovereignty, Effectiveness, and Legitimacy in a Transnational Order," in *Complex Sovereignty: Reconstituting Political Authority in the Twenty-First Century*, eds. Edgar Grande and Louis W. Pauly (Toronto: University of Toronto Press, 2005), 5–6; John Gerard Ruggie, "Reconstituting the Global Public Domain: Issues, Actors, and Practices" (Faculty Research Working Paper Series, JFK School of Government, Harvard University, July 2004), 1.

7.   See Katherine Sikkink and Jackie Smith, "Infrastructure for Change: Transnational Organizations, 1953–93," in *Restructuring World Politics: Transnational Social Movements, Networks, and Norms*, eds. Sanjeev Khagram, James V. Riker, and Kathryn Sikkink (Minneapolis: University of Minnesota Press, 2002), 24–46. The term *global governance* (in contrast to *transnational governance*), if taken literally, is often an exaggeration or aspiration that assumes or expects that the nation-state has been or will be eclipsed in authority by other international actors. More often it is used to refer to any process or relationship that crosses state borders: "The term 'transnational' is in a way more humble, and offers a more adequate label for phenomena which can be quite variable in scale and distribution, even when they share the characteristic of not being contained within the state." Ulf Hannerz, *Transnational Connections: Culture, People, Places* (London: Routledge, 1996), 6.

8.   See Gill Walt and Kent Buse, "Global Cooperation in International Public Health," in *International Public Health: Diseases, Programs, Systems, and Policies*, eds. Michael H. Merson, Robert E. Black, and Anne J. Mills, (Sudbury, MA: Jones and Bartlett, 2006), 649–80.

9.   Health governance refers to "the actions and means adopted by a society to organize itself in the promotion and protection of the health of its population." Richard Dodgson, Kelley Lee, and Nick

alliances, global health partnerships, and global public-private partnerships in health, to name a few.[10]

At a deep level, the forces of globalization and the emergence of old and new infectious diseases have driven this process of institutional and policy adaptation.[11] Economic integration, urbanization, and technological advancement that permits expanded international travel and transport coupled with the fact that many health issues "circumvent, undermine, or are oblivious to the territorial boundaries of states and, thus, beyond the capacity of states to address effectively through state institutions alone," have compelled new, transnational efforts.[12]

At a more mundane level, various factors have abetted this process of governance, especially changing ideological and institutional preferences and new sources of funding.[13] The emergence of neoliberal ideologies in public policymaking in the 1980s, first in the United States and Great Britain and later in international organizations, encouraged and legitimized new forms of linkages between the public and private sectors in the search for creative ideas and greater efficiency in governance. Concomitantly, some states became increasingly disillusioned with the United Nations and its agencies by that time.[14] In health, for example, several governments and analysts expressed concerns over the WHO's bureaucratic procedures, costs, lack of budgetary transparency, and inability to determine priorities. These attitudes, and relatively stagnant economic growth in the 1970s and 1980s, led governments to reduce in real terms their financial support for the general budget of the United Nations and some of its agencies and to increase their financial support for specialized and supplemental budgets earmarked for new public-private initiatives.

Drager, *Global Health Governance: A Conceptual Review* (Geneva: World Health Organization and London School of Hygiene and Tropical Medicine, 2002).

10. See Mark W. Zacher and Tania J. Keefe, *The Politics of Global Health Governance: United by Contagion* (New York: Palgrave Macmillan, 2008).

11. See Anne Marie Kimball et al., "Regional Infectious Disease Surveillance Networks and Their Potential to Facilitate the Implementation of the International Health Regulations," *Medical Clinics North America* 92 (2008): 1459–71.

12. Kelley Lee, Suzanne Fustukian, and Kent Buse, "An Introduction to Global Health Policy," in *Health Policy in a Globalising World*, ed. Kelley Lee, Susan Fustukian, and Kent Buse (Cambridge: Cambridge University Press, 2002), 3–17.

13. Rene Loewenson, "Civil Society Influence on Global Health Policy" (online report, Geneva: World Health Organization, 2003), www.tarsc.org/WHOCSI/globalhealth.php. See also Marco Schaferhoff, Sabine Campe, and Christopher Kaan, "Transnational Public-Private Partnerships in International Relations: Making Sense of Concepts, Research Frameworks, and Results," *International Studies Review* 11, no. 3 (September 2009): 451–74.

14. Walt and Buse, "Global Cooperation," 663.

In time, the United Nations and the UN family of organizations, following the lead of international organizations such as the World Bank, adapted to this new reality. The UN secretary-general came to embrace the notion of "global compact of shared values and principles"[15] between the public and private sectors, as did many UN agencies.[16] In health, WHO adopted this idea in earnest by the mid-1990s, asserting that through partnerships "we can enhance significantly our ability to mobilize, social, political, and therefore, financial support for health development and international health cooperation."[17] WHO director Gro Harlem Brundtland urged the WHO to aggressively pursue partnerships with the private sector noting that "in a world filed with complex health problems, WHO cannot solve them alone. Governments cannot solve them alone. Nongovernmental organizations, the private sector, and foundations cannot solve them alone. Only through new and innovative partnerships can we make a difference. Whether we like it or not, we are dependent on the partners . . . to bridge the gap and achieve health for all."[18] Furthermore, WHO's IHR 2005 added another normative endorsement of public-private partnerships in disease surveillance as it encouraged governments to participate in international networks as part of their surveillance strategy and to improve global outbreak intelligence.[19]

New sources of public funding and new private philanthropic giving in health engaged the participation of private nongovernmental organizations, which saw public-private partnerships as a way to further their public health agendas. National governments also increasingly looked beyond their respective health ministries for service enhancements that could be provided by private business and NGOs. As a result, health-related NGOs proliferated at both the country and international level. For corporations, private-public partnerships in health afforded both an opportunity for policy influence and a means of effectively responding to calls for greater corporate responsibility and citizenship. In a more attenuated sense, corporate involvement in partnerships also opened up potential avenues to new markets and products.

In sum, transnational public-private policy networks have grown in number, issue, scope, and importance.[20] They also assume a variety of forms, serve

---

15. Kent Buse and Gill Walt, "Global Public-Private Partnerships: Part I, A New Development in Health," *Bulletin of the World Health Organization* 78, no. 4 (2000): 8.

16. Judith Richter, "Public-Private Partnerships for Health: A Trend with No Alternatives," *Development* 47, no. 2 (2004): 43–48.

17. Buse and Walt, "Global Public-Private Partnerships," 9.

18. Richter, "Public-Private Partnerships," 44.

19. Kimball et al., "Regional Infectious Disease," 1461.

20. For a good summary, see Edgar Grande and Louis W. Pauly, "Complex Sovereignty and the Emergence of Transnational Authority," in *Complex Sovereignty: Reconstituting Political Authority in the*

a variety of purposes, and are active in the area of public health. With the rise of this new form of governance have come questions about its effectiveness, legitimacy, and organizational processes. Detailed analysis of the governance process in these three cases provides a basis for systematic comparison and an opportunity to distill meaningful hypotheses and generalizations about these new transnational organizations both for scholars interested in the relationship among states, nongovernmental organizations, transnational corporations, and international organizations in international governance, and for practitioners and policy makers engaged in addressing transnational problems in varied contexts.

The Great Debates

In the growing academic literature on transnational public-private partnerships (PPPs), two fundamental questions dominate. First is whether transnational PPPs are effective in devising and delivering cooperative solutions to pressing transnational problems. If they are successful, what factors contribute to their ability to craft and implement cooperative policy solutions and, conversely, to the extent they do not achieve their aims, what factors impede their effectiveness? This line of inquiry requires specifying what constitutes success for these networks.[21] Second, are the networks legitimate and accountable in their exercise of political authority? Here too, we want to know what factors contribute to legitimacy (defined how?), and accountability (to whom?), and what factors impede legitimacy and accountability.[22]

Proponents of transnational PPPs see them as filling a gap in governance and responding to the limitations of both states and markets in meeting international challenges by pooling different resources, skills, and expertise to provide collective goods.[23] For example, foundations and corporations often

Twenty-First Century, eds. Edgar Grande and Louis W. Pauly (Toronto: University of Toronto Press, 2005), 285–300.

21. See, for example, Michael R. Reich, ed., *Public-Private Partnerships for Public Health*, Harvard Series on Population and International Health (Cambridge, MA: Harvard Center for Population and Development Studies, April 2002); Schaferhoff, Campe, and Kaan, "Transnational Public-Private Partnerships," 451–74.

22. Grande and Pauly, "Complex Sovereignty," 293; Schaferhoff, Campe, and Kaan, "Transnational Public-Private Partnerships," 451; Tania A. Borzel and Thomas Risse, "Public-Private Partnerships: Effective and Legitimate Tools of Transnational Governance," in *Complex Sovereignty: Reconstituting Political Authority in the Twenty-First Century*, eds. Edgar Grande and Louis W. Pauly (Toronto: University of Toronto Press, 2005), 195–216.

23. For a good discussion of the various strengths of the respective public and private actors in transnational governance, see Pauline Vaillancourt Rosenau, "The Strengths and Weaknesses of Public-Private Policy Partnerships," in *Public-Private Policy Partnerships*, ed. Pauline Vaillancourt Rosenau (Cambridge, MA: MIT Press, 2000), 217–42.

bring substantial material resources, and INGOs and NGOs bring expertise, local knowledge, and sometimes moral authority to their partnerships with governments and international organizations. The motivation of the various actors is not necessarily to fill governmental gaps, per se. Rather, by pursuing interests in partnership that they could not secure acting alone or through existing intergovernmental arrangements, they effectively perform governance functions. This effectiveness in problem solving and delivery of public goods is sometimes equated with the output legitimacy of transnational PPPs.[24] In public health, the argument is often made that neither governments nor earlier systems of intergovernmental cooperation is adequate in meeting today's policy challenges in the face of globalization, which increases both the number of risks to health and the speed at which such risks travel.[25]

Furthermore, advocates maintain that transnational PPPs increase the legitimacy (defined as democratic accountability) of international governance because they expand the number and types of actors involved in governance to include INGOs, TNCs, and transnational social movements, strengthening so-called input legitimacy by making policy and institutions accountable to more and more divergent stakeholders.[26] This feature of transnational PPPs also reinforces their output legitimacy (effectiveness). The argument is that by including more of the so-called rule targets in the process of rule-making, transnational PPPs help ensure greater likelihood of compliance with international norms and rules.[27] Input legitimacy is further enhanced, advocates say, by the deliberative quality and consensual decision-making processes that characterize transnational PPPs.[28] More often than not, decisions are reached by reasoned consensus rather than majority vote over a bargained compromise. Arguably, the process of consensus building leads to better problem solving and mutual learning and can, in theory, play an important role in breaking down stereotypical views

24. See, for example, Fritz W. Scharpf, "Introduction: The Problem-Solving Capacity of Multi-level Governance," *Journal of European Public Policy* 4 (1997): 520–38.

25. Sarah Payne, "Globalization, Governance, and Health," in *Governance, Globalization and Public Policy*, ed. Patricia Kennett (Cheltenham, UK: Edward Elgar, 2008), 151–72.

26. A central principle of democratic theory is that leaders and government must be held accountable for their actions. "In democratic systems, a social order is legitimate because the rulers are accountable to their citizens who can participate in the rule-making through representation, and can punish the rulers by voting them out of office." Risse, "Transnational Governance and Legitimacy," 6.

27. Abram Chayes, Antonia Handler Chayes, and Ronald B. Mitchell, "Managing Compliance: A Comparative Perspective," in *Engaging Countries: Strengthening Compliance with International Environmental Accords*, eds. Edith Brown Weiss and Harold K. Jacobsen (Cambridge, MA: MIT Press, 1998), 39–62.

28. Risse, "Transnational Governance and Legitimacy."

of different actors and opening up possibilities for improved coordination among organizations.[29]

Skeptics criticize transnational PPPs as ineffective in delivering public goods to the public[30] and for serving primarily the interests of commercial and private parties.[31] Most of this criticism is directed toward corporate-government-intergovernmental efforts such as the Global Fund to Fight AIDS, Tuberculosis, and Malaria, but the same brush has tarred INGO-facilitated partnerships, like the ones studied here. Critics often suggest that transnational PPPs have a deleterious effect on the provision of public goods by allowing states to abdicate their responsibility for public goods delivery or diverting resources away from state priorities, and fragmenting and confusing the policy landscape so that international governmental organizations cannot effectively devise global solutions.[32] If international organizations such as the UN are denied resources and authority is delegated to nonstate actors, the result, critics claim, is "problem shifting" rather than "problem solving"[33] and the erosion of public competence.[34] With regard to public health, Kent Buse and Gill Walt write that transnational PPPs "may lead to the further weakening of the U.N. system," and "may undermine the ability of the WHO to effectively contribute to health governance at a global level"[35] and undermine the U.N. aims for cooperation and equity among states.[36] The involvement of more and more actors with divergent interests and values does not enhance problem solving, as proponents maintain, but produces lowest common denominator solutions or stalemates.[37]

Critics also challenge the inclusiveness and input legitimacy of transnational PPPs because they grant nonstate actors the opportunity to engage

---

29. Ronald W. McQuaid, "The Theory of Partnerships. Why Have Partnerships?" in *Public-Private Partnerships: Theory and Practice in International Perspective*, ed. Stephen P. Osborne (London: Routledge, 2000), 9–35.

30. Renate Mayntz notes, "By definition, governance refers to the solution of *collective* problems and the production of *public* welfare." "From Government to Governance," 7.

31. See, for example, Kent Buse and Gill Walt, "Globalisation and Multilateral Public-Private Health Partnerships: Issues for Health Policy," in *Health Policy in a Globalising World*, eds. Kelley Lee, Susan Fustukian, and Kent Buse (Cambridge: Cambridge University Press, 2002), 4–62; Richter, "Public-Private Partnerships," 46.

32. See, for example, Sania Nishtar, "Public-Private 'Partnerships' in Health—A Global Call to Action," *Health Policy Research and Systems* 2, no. 5 (2004): 5–11, www.health-policy-systems.com/content/2/1/5.

33. Borzel and Risse, "Public-Private Partnerships," 209.

34. Buse and Walt, "Globalisation and Multilateral," 57.

35. Ibid., 42.

36. Kent Buse and Gill Walt, "The World Health Organization and Global Public-Private Health Partnerships: In Search of Good Global Governance," in *Public-Private Partnerships: Theory and Practice in International Perspective*, ed. Stephen P. Osborne (London: Routledge, 2000), 169–96.

37. Schaferhoff, Campe, and Kaan, "Transnational Public-Private Partnerships," 459.

in authoritative decision making. Some fear that by including private-sector actors in policymaking, especially TNCs, private commercial interests will de facto control or manipulate public policy by virtue of the superior resources they bring to the partnerships: those who pay the piper will call the tune.[38] Similarly, some see transnational PPPs as reinforcing power asymmetries in the international system because the actors, including INGO participants, are overwhelmingly elites from wealthy nations with similar, Western values.[39] One set of writers refers to this characteristic of transnational PPPs as "elite pluralism."[40]

Although there is no shortage of opinion about transnational PPPs, there is a dearth of evidence about their effectiveness, legitimacy, and internal operations. Tanya Borzel's and Thomas Risse's survey of the literature concludes, "little empirical evidence is available on PPPs and their influence on [policy effectiveness and legitimacy], and the evidence that is available is often selective and compiled in such a way as to limit its analytical value. . . . We need to know a lot more about the inter- as well as the intra-organizational dynamics of transnational PPPs."[41] These authors also remind us to be explicit about the yardsticks against which we measure the effectiveness and legitimacy of transnational PPPs. By effectiveness, do we refer to the ability of transnational PPPs to follow procedural norms, produce outputs, or deliver problem-solving outcomes? With regard to legitimacy, do we expect transnational PPPs to meet the ideals of cosmopolitan democracy[42] or are international governmental organizations and interstate regimes the appropriate standard for assessing transnational PPPs?[43]

In the next section, I consider the issue of the effectiveness and legitimacy of these transnational infectious disease surveillance networks and highlight from the cases the key variables associated with their performance in these two respects. This chapter also discusses hypotheses about the origins

---

38. Kent Buse and Andrew Harmer, "Power to the Partners? The Politics of Public-Private Health Partnerships," *Development* 47, no. 2 (2004): 49–56.

39. Ibid.

40. Kent Buse et al., "Globalisation and Health Policy: Trends and Opportunities," in *Health Policy in a Globalising World*, eds. Kelley Lee, Susan Fustukian, and Kent Buse (Cambridge: Cambridge University Press, 2002), 251–80.

41. Borzel and Risse, "Public-Private Partnerships," 196, 213. Similarly, as Michael Reich explains in the introduction of *Public-Private Partnerships for Public Health*, "we know so little about the conditions where partnerships succeed" (Cambridge, MA: Harvard Center for Population and Development Studies, April 2002), 2.

42. This is the standard recommended in Carmen Hackel Schneider, "Global Public Health and International Relations: Pressing Issues—Evolving Governance," *Australian Journal of International Affairs* 62, no. 1 (March 2008): 94–106.

43. This standard is recommended in Schaferhoff, Campe, and Kaan, "Transnational Public-Private Partnerships," 469. See also Borzel and Risse, "Public-Private Partnerships," 213–14.

of transnational PPPs and their relationship with states and international organizations for further study.

Effectiveness of Transnational PPPs: Lessons from Networks

Effective transnational governance in policy formulation and implementation and the delivery of services depends first on the willingness and ability of states to cooperate in these new institutional arrangements.[44] Chapter 3 has already assessed the ability of member states in two of the three organizations (MBDS and MECIDS) to overcome historic antipathies, asymmetries of power among the membership, insufficient domestic capacity in some members, and divergent political ideas and policy preferences, to achieve a very high level of cooperation.[45] Interstate cooperation, along with the participation and support of private actors and international organizations, has led to effectiveness in public good production in both MBDS and MECIDS and to much less effectiveness in the case of EAIDSNet.

To summarize the insights from chapter 3, the three critical components of interstate cooperation within transnational public-private partnership are as follows:

Shared interest among the states in a valuable transnational public good. If the sought-after transnational public good carries with it consumption externalities, and if failure to secure the particular common goods results in profound state vulnerability to a transnational threat, so much the better.

Appropriate membership in the new transnational entity to include all states with a meaningful stake in securing the public good and to exclude those states and other international actors that are extraneous to the group's success. Members should be able to act authoritatively for their home governments both in setting goals and implementing decisions.

Regular, personal, productive contact among the key actors to breakdown existing oppositional identities, and to redefine the in-group to include the full membership of the new transnational organization. Trust must be built among the principal actors and within the larger institution structure.

In additional to these components of interstate cooperation, the cases reveal several other factors that contribute to the effectiveness of a transnational PPP. First, the transnational PPP should be in compliance with and

---

44. Policy formulation relates to the development of norms, rules, and standards that are designed to regulate state behavior and policy implementation refers to the actual implementation of these policies and delivery of support to targeted populations. Schaferhoff, Campe, and Kaan, "Transnational Public-Private Partnerships," 457.

45. Grande and Pauly, "Complex Sovereignty," 293–95.

in the furtherance of existing international norms,[46] and in support of and congruent with the activities of international organizations operating in the policy space.[47] Congruence with international norms has two salutary effects: it strengthens the international norm, and it adds an element of moral obligation and the possibility of international opprobrium to calculations of state self-interest, thereby contributing to compliance by state actors with the decisions of the transnational PPP.[48]

Transnational networks such as MBDS and MECIDS have reinforced international compliance with international disease surveillance norms, principles, and standards embodied in the WHO's IHR 2005 and with the workings of related global efforts in disease reporting such as ProMED-mail. By applying and enhancing these international standards at a subregional level, MBDS and MECIDS increase compliance with global norms and practices and extend these standards for performance. The policies and practices of these two networks raise the baseline global standard for infectious disease surveillance, reporting, and response and contextualize the IHR 2005. Practically, their actions also make international norms and aspirations for global health more effective because, in emphasizing local problems, regional PPPs combat infectious diseases before those diseases become global threats. This is not to suggest that all international civil servants at the WHO or all health scholars are happy with the loss of monopolistic control over disease surveillance and response by international organizations represented by these emerging transnational PPPs.[49] But this aspiration for a UN system that does everything centrally is anachronistic, controlling, and ultimately detrimental to effective disease control at both the regional and the global level.

Second, transnational public-private networks should strengthen the core capacities of each of its members and of the network as a whole. In this way, transnational networks empower, rather than absolve, states of fulfilling their responsibility to deliver public health goods to their populations and they enhance, not diminish, the abilities of fragile national public systems (in health). The four critical capabilities in infectious disease control are establishing common laboratory standards and procedures; improving disease detection and joint outbreak investigation and response; standardizing

46.   Risse, "Transnational Governance and Legitimacy," 15.
47.   Nishtar, "Public-Private 'Partnerships' in Health," 5–11; Buse and Harmer, "Power to the Partners," 49–56.
48.   Ian Hurd, "Legitimacy and Authority," 387.
49.   See, for example, Buse and Harmer, "Power to the Partners," 49–56; Phillipe Calain, "Exploring the International Arena of Global Public Health Surveillance," *Health Policy and Planning* 22, no. 1 (2007): 2–12.

reporting mechanisms and increasing the speed and frequency of intelligence; and training personnel in essential skills and knowledge bases (such as field epidemiology and information systems) and promoting joint scientific research. The operations of the MBDS and MECIDS networks and the activities of EAIDSNet and the EAC Health Sector have reinforced operational competence at the national level and upgraded the infectious disease surveillance systems and public health core competencies in each country participant. In the cases of MBDS and MECIDS, the overall capacities of the networks have grown over time.[50] Both have made substantial strides in improving the core capacities of their members, both individually and collectively, whereas in East Africa integration of regional cooperation has made less progress relative to the strengthening of individual national systems.[51]

Third, effective transnational PPPs should leverage the strengths of the partners by ensuring that they play roles within the organization that are appropriate to their strengths.[52] What are these roles? Broadly defined, the role of states is to create a political and legal environment conducive to joint policy making and joint and severable policy implementation. The participation of private firms and philanthropies are primarily for the generation of wealth, material resources, and sometimes expertise. Civil and international NGOs facilitate social and political interaction by convening, mobilizing, advising, and cajoling key actors and drawing on their expertise, moral authority, and network of contacts. International organizations should set global norms and frameworks for action and provide resources in the form of financial support, coordination, and expertise. The respective roles are not dictates, of course, but to the extent that actors do not play to their strengths, transnational PPPs will be less effective and, as discussed below, less legitimate as well. In the cases of MBDS and MECIDS, the correspondence between the archetypical roles of actors in a transnational PPP and the actual role of the partner organizations is strong.

Fourth, the right balance between formality and flexibility is critical. Clearly, the existence of concrete plans, monitoring progress toward goals, and assigning well-defined responsibilities, together with unambiguous, achievable goals, contributed to the effectiveness of MBDS and MECIDS.[53] Both organizations, for example, set out and published multiyear plans of operation with specific goals rather than articulating vague aspirations. They

---

50. Kimball et al., "Regional Infectious Disease."
51. See chapter 2.
52. Rosenau, "Strengths and Weaknesses," 219; Buse et al., "Globalisation and Health Policy," 260.
53. Rosenau, "Strengths and Weaknesses," 232.

Figure 3. Effectiveness of Transnational Public-Private Partnerships

Necessary Condition	Facilitating Factors
Interstate cooperation via • shared interest in a transnational public good • membership that includes all and only relevant actors • creation of a new in-group identity through decategorization and recategorization and building trust through personal, protracted, positive contact	• congruence with international norms and activities of IGOs • strengthening core capacities of membership individually and collectively • appropriate roles for actors that play to their respective organizational strengths • formality of plans, goals, responsibility that allows for flexibility and adaptability • committed founding donors and multiple revenue streams

also apportioned responsibility for achieving particular goals. The MBDS strategic plan of 2008–2013, with its seven strategic initiatives and individual country representatives appointed to lead each initiative, is a good illustration. Effectiveness in transnational governance is an art, not a science, however. So, although plans, goals, and responsibilities are important, so too is operational flexibility and adaptability. We also can see evidence of these qualities in MBDS and MECIDS. For example, the two organizations differ in the formality of their founding constitutional documents. MBDS is more public and official, and uses intergovernmental MOUs. MECIDS, befitting the political sensitivities in the region, is less formal and uses no foundational document (members like to joke that the organization does not exist). This variability is a strength rather than a weakness of the two organizations. Also, as noted, these two networks and EAIDSNet were not subject to precise, politically determined deadlines or benchmarks. This flexibility, especially in their formative period, allowed them to begin a process of building trust without undue haste or scrutiny. Likewise, MBDS and MECIDS, though they have precise plans, have been able to adapt both plans and priorities to changing circumstances and needs. We can see this quality in their rapid response to potentially pandemic avian influenza and their ability to incorporate this acute problem into their programs.

A fifth and final factor contributing to the effectiveness of transnational PPPs is multiple revenue streams and dedicated supporters. The two most successful regional infectious disease networks had core founding supporters (the Rockefeller Foundation and the Global Health and Security Initiative of NTI) and funding from numerous other partners drawn from the ranks of international organizations (the Asian Development Bank and World Bank), foundations (Gates and Google), and private corporations (IBM and Becton Dickson). In contrast, EAIDSNet struggled in its efforts to diversify its sources of funding. Unable to secure multiple revenue streams, EAIDSNet was compelled to find a different institutional arrangement for its programs. For a summary of the necessary and facilitating factors for effective transnational public-private partnership, see figure 3.

Transnational PPPs: Lessons from Networks

What makes a transnational PPP legitimate? Here I refer to input legitimacy, the democratic quality of the decision making processes of transnational PPPs. This quality is in contrast to their output legitimacy, that is, their ability to solve problems and accomplish stated goals, already discussed under the rubric of effectiveness.[54] Democratic decision making means that those affected by collective decisions are represented and provide meaningful input into an inclusive decision-making process.[55] Because the members of a transnational PPP are not typically elected directly by popular consent, their democratic legitimacy in the case studies (and in most other instances) is indirect and comes from two sources. First, the decision-making power of state participants is an extension, by delegation, of state authority that allows state actors to participate legitimately in the transnational organization. In the last resort, their populations (or whomever claims state sovereignty) may hold the state participants responsible for the activities of the transnational organization. Second, the participation of international and civil nongovernmental groups and TNCs generally accepted as legitimate in their defined sphere of activity can, by their participation with states, make transnational organizations more inclusive, for example, in comparison with purely intergovernmental organizations.[56] As noted, some critics find the delegation of decision-making authority to a transnational public-private entity an attenuated form of democratic legitimacy and believe that some private actors (corporations) are, by their nature, illegitimate in public policymaking. By this standard, few national governments would qualify as democratically accountable either.

In MBDS, MECIDS, and EAIDSNet, the decision makers were primarily state representatives to the transnational PPP. Their legitimacy is by virtue of delegation from their respective states and no different than their participation in an intergovernmental organization. In fact, because they include all and only the state actors immediately affected by its

54. Of course, from a purely consequentialist perspective, if a transnational PPP is effective, it is, necessarily, legitimate.

55. Schäferhoff, Campe, and Kaan, "Transnational Public-Private Partnerships," 466.

56. Grande and Pauly, "Complex Sovereignty," 297.

decisions, and not, for example, more powerful but less affected northern states, these three organizations are more directly democratic than a global IGO, in which the interest of the richest and most powerful countries, rather than the most affected, are more likely to dominate. The global climate change discussion illustrates well how the voices of the most affected populations (islanders) can be lost in a large gathering of more powerful states. MBDS and MECIDS also included a variety of private partners, but their roles, though important and essential, were secondary to state actors who made the critical decisions and set the strategic direction of the organization. In this sense, these two organizations were more inclusive in reaching out to private actors to leverage available resources and expertise without unduly privatizing public policy.

Participation is one measure of meaningful democratic practice, equitably exercising power is yet another. In assessing the legitimacy of transnational governance structures, Jim Whitman wonders, "Where is power in this picture?"[57] and Kent Buse and Andrew Harmer ask, "Who has power, how is power exercised, and on what basis?"[58] In searching for the locus of power in transnational PPPs, Buse and Harmer direct us to investigate the composition of the paramount decision-making board, the membership criterion, and the hosting arrangements.[59]

The board membership of both MBDS and MECIDS includes one to three official state representatives of each country participant, each with equal voting weight, and the board chair rotates among members on an annual basis. Decision making in both MBDS and MECIDS is conducted on the basis of strict equality and decisions are made by deliberation and unanimous board consensus. Private actors facilitate and support the board and its programs, but do not have a direct decision-making role. This is not to say that in its operations, each national actor has identical infectious-disease-fighting capacity in terms of diagnostic or information systems and plays an identical role in the implementation of policies. In this operational sense, equity and interoperability of systems, rather than strict equality, are the guiding norms. Each country has its own public health system through which the recommendations of the transnational entity must be interpreted and implemented. Operationally, the organizations emphasize improving the capacities of its weaker members, but also take

57. Jim Whitman, "Global Governance as the Friendly Face of Unaccountable Power," *Security Dialogue* 33, no. 1 (2002): 47.

58. Buse and Harmer, "Power to the Partners," 49.

59. Ibid., 53–55.

advantage of the particular capabilities of its strongest members so as to avoid redundancies and inefficiencies.

Hosting arrangements are also sensitive to the need to share responsibilities and opportunities equitably among membership. As described in chapter 2, MECIDS has two homes for its secretariat, one in East Jerusalem and one in Amman. Its board meets in different localities, including nonmember states, because these neutral sites can be easier for obtaining travel visas and accommodating its members. MBDS has a single secretariat, in Bangkok, but its board meetings rotate among the member states, which often meet in key border-crossing zones. In is early years, EAIDSNet rotated the site of its meetings and moved them to border districts to be closer to the populations at greatest risk.

Accountability is a third factor contributing to legitimacy. It refers to the question of who is entitled to control the decision makers and participants in a transnational PPP. Which external audiences will review and approve policies? Accountability has two dimensions, internal and external. Internal accountability refers to authorization of principals to agents who are institutionally linked to one another. More simply, it means the accountability one has to the party that put one in a position of responsibility. Examples include the accountability of health ministers or public health directors to their home governments or cabinets; the accountability of corporate actors to their CEO, shareholders, customers, or watchdog organizations; and NGO accountability to their boards of directors and contributors. External accountability refers to the accountability of actors to those affected by their actions. In the case of infectious disease control networks, this would mean those whose health is impacted by the decisions of the transnational PPP.[60]

Because of the many MBDS and MECIDS stakeholders, there are numerous loci of internal accountability. Each actor, whether from the governmental, corporate, or nonprofit sector, has its own accountability mechanism or mechanisms. For the transnational PPP to be successful over time, it must satisfy all these masters. In some respects, one could argue that transnational PPPs have to serve too many constituencies. Nonetheless, the participants in MBDS and MECIDS have acquitted themselves to those who entrusted them, whereas EAIDSNet experienced difficulty in sustaining buy-in from all its constituents.

External accountability in this instance would refer primarily to the public health of the populations affected by the decisions of the transnational

---

60. Robert Keohane, "Accountability in World Politics," *Scandinavian Political Studies* 29, no. 2 (2006): 75–87.

entities. Here, accountability is indirect, through governmental account-ability mechanisms in each member state. In addition, each member state, with the exception of the Palestinian Authority, is accountable to WHO in meeting the standards set by IHR 2005.

Individuals affected by the public-private policies of MBDS and MEC-IDS have some indirect say in the operation of these organizations, more so, I would suggest, than they might at most intergovernmental organiza-tions or in other issue areas. This argument rests on three points. First, each organization gathers data and inputs directly from the affected populations in the form of both health reports and local concerns and advice garnered at various community meetings. In this sense, they have a grassroots con-nection to those individuals and localities they are trying to serve. Second, as regional bodies, or more accurately, as subregional organizations, they are more directly accountable for their decisions and actions than many larger regional or global organizations, in which the interests of the affected popu-lations must often compete with the interests of actors whose populations are less affected. Finally, health impacts are measurable and comparable, so to the extent the facts are reported (see the discussion of transparency that follows), they constitute a clear metric by which to hold these transnational organizations and their member states accountable to the populations they are designed to serve.

A critical condition for both internal and external accountability is trans-parency. Are the agendas, agreements, activities, and assessments of the transnational PPP available to the public? MBDS, MECIDS, and (in its early years) EAIDSNet receive good marks for transparency. The trans-national organizations themselves publish their minutes, agreements, and strategic plans on the Internet. Usually they make these items available in a timely fashion. Outcomes are shared through newsletters and their Web sites. Detailed health metrics and the implementation steps taken by each member state are less available and remain primarily the responsibility of states to report. Also, the various partners, state and nonstate, typically pub-lish annual reports and newsletters that share information about the net-work's activities. To a limited extent, the public media occasionally report on these organizations. It is not clear whether the lack of independent media coverage is attributable to the technical nature of the issue or to the desire of the transnational PPPs to shield themselves from greater publicity that could constrain their actions, create political problems in some of the home states, or create runaway expectations for peace among the public.

Figure 4. Legitimacy and Accountability of Transnational Public-Private Partnerships

Inclusive participation

Equitable exercise of power in
- membership criteria
- leadership and the decision-making board
- hosting functions

Significant and multiple loci of accountability of each actor
- to those that delegated them authority
- to affected populations

Transparency of organization structure, decision-making processes, and programs
- publications and promulgations of the transnational network
- publications and promulgations of the individual members of the transnational network
- openness to public media

Deliberative and consensual decisionmaking

Finally, the democratic legitimacy of transnational PPPs can be enhanced through the deliberative quality of the decision-making process and the ability of the organization to achieve a reasoned consensus rather than a bargaining compromise.[61] The decision-making processes of MBDS and MECIDS are based on consensus, unanimity, and strict equality and vividly illustrate this point. These decision-making norms not only enhance democratic legitimacy, they also build trust and reflect the mutual respect so important to building cooperation among actors that do not have a history of effective collaboration. Figure 4 summarizes the factors that contribute to the legitimacy and accountability of transnational public-private networks.

Origins and External Relations of Transnational PPPs

This study also affords an opportunity to raise questions about the origins and external relationships of transnational public-private partnerships that warrant further investigation. The first issue concerns the origins of transnational PPPs. Are they the inspiration of affected polities and publics, or do policy entrepreneurs from wealthy governments or organizations instigate them? Do subregional health networks, in particular, arise as a response to a health crisis or gaps in governance as seen from the bottom up or the top down? The answer suggested by the three case studies is complicated and equivocal. In the case of MBDS, the inspiration came from the Rockefeller Foundation and a small group of public health officials from some of the member states. In East Africa, the public health officials from the three

---

61. Risse, "Transnational Governance and Legitimacy," 16.

states had an initial plan to address malaria outbreak that they later broadened to include a more comprehensive list of infectious diseases to match the interests of a private foundation. In the case of MECIDS, it was the inspiration of two private actors—an INGO and a foundation—to launch a regional public-private partnership in a regional security issue, but it was the health officials of the states who steered this aspiration toward the issue of infectious disease control.

The cases suggest two observations. First, foundations, by virtue of their bird's eye view of transnational problems and their financial and reputational powers to convene and network are ideal instigators for the creation of transnational public-private partnerships. Second, launching a public-private partnership requires quick uptake by ready, willing, and able state actors. As noted in chapter 3, it is the overlapping of public and private interests and a shared belief that actors are more likely to realize their interests together rather than apart that lays the foundation for new transnational PPPs.

Second, this study allows us to consider the relationship between these horizontally organized networks with hierarchical states—are they collaborators, substitutes, or opponents? Similarly, we can ask, "How do these regional networks relate to international architectures—are they complementary or competitive? With regard to the first issue, the answer is clear. Effective transnational public-private partnerships must collaborate with states; they can neither usurp state authority nor operate in opposition to it. Although state participants forgo a measure of national sovereignty to join a transnational PPP, their sovereign powers and legitimate claims to authority are indispensable to the success of hybrid governance. With regard to the second issue, transnational PPPs in this study for the most part complemented and reinforced the norms, rules, and standards set by intergovernmental organizations. By the same token, though, elements of competition between PPPs and intergovernmental organizations exist, as do both issues of redundancy and lack of coordination in this policy space. MBDS and MECIDS generally worked in sync with multilateral bodies. In the case of EAIDSNet, other intergovernmental initiatives served to distract participants from building cross-border collaboration. Transnational PPPs in infectious disease control are new policy actors. More senior international bodies therefore view them with a mixture of appreciation, admiration, and suspicion. These subregional entities share jurisdiction with a larger regional body, such as ASEAN in the case of MBDS, and with global actors such as the WHO and WHO-supported global initiatives. It is difficult to know, much less efficiently manage, all the infectious disease control initiatives at a particular place and time.

Conclusion: Hypotheses on Transnational Governance

Transnational public-private partnerships take on too many forms and perform too many functions to issue definitive conclusions about what makes them effective and legitimate, where they come from, or how they best function relative to traditional state actors and intergovernmental organizations. This comparative study does allow us to suggest several theoretical propositions, however. With regard to effectiveness, it suggests that interstate cooperation is an indispensable element for effective transnational PPPs. Chapter 3 discusses in detail the three components—interests, institutions, and identities—that must align for interstate cooperation in transnational PPPs, especially in situations that involve state actors without a strong history of cooperation. As discussed in this chapter, the cases indicate other factors can contribute to the effective operation of transnational PPP, when effectiveness means actual problem solving or remediation and the delivery of an essential public good (the highest standard for effectiveness). These salutary factors include the following items:

- congruence with international norms and the practice of international organizations;
- policies that strengthen the capacity of each member and the partnership as a whole;
- partnership roles that correspond to the particular strengths and capacities of the actors involved;
- formal plans and concrete goals and responsibilities, but not arbitrary or politically inspired timetables so as to allow for some flexibility and adaptability in programs and procedures; and
- a committed core and multiple auxiliary sources of financial supporters.

The cases also suggest that the key variables contributing to the legitimacy of transnational PPPs defined in terms of democratic accountability include the following:

- inclusive membership to allow for voice by many parties with a stake in the outcome of decisions;
- the equitable exercise of power as reflected in the key institutions and internal rules of the transnational organization;

- accountability of all parties to one or preferably several empowering authorities and affected populations;
- organizational transparency ideally from multiple sources of reporting (the transnational PPP itself, the members of the PPP, and independent sources such as media); and
- deliberative and consensual decision making.

The cases are not so numerous as to suggest which of these factors carries greatest weight in the process of legitimating transnational PPPs.

It appears that states acting at the urging or with the early support of a private actor with resources (ideational or financial or both) are the pas de deux for launching a transnational PPP initiative. The notion of transnational initiative sustaining itself from a single organization or perspective—be it north or south, grass roots or elite—seems unlikely, however, because it is the overlapping of interests and interdependence among actors that characterizes this form of transnational relationship.

Finally, the cases suggest that transnational PPPs do not imply a withering away of the state or that transnational forms of governance have superseded state sovereignty. Rather, states remain the most important and the indispensable partner in transnational arrangements even as these new arrangements are a departure from the idealized Westphalian model of state monopoly over sovereignty. The relationship is complex. Generally, these new entities complement the work of intergovernmental organizations rather than confound them. At the same time, they add a new player to international policymaking process and this addition brings with it new opportunities and ideas on the one hand, and new challenges of accommodation and coordination with purely intergovernmental bodies on the other.

5

PANDEMIC PREEMPTION: U.S. FOREIGN POLICY IN SUPPORT OF OVERSEAS CAPACITY

In addition to the emerging subregional networks of cooperation focused on in earlier chapters and the pan-regional and global organizations noted in chapter 2, the public health policies of states also play a critical role in the fight against pandemics. This chapter examines in detail the policy of a key national actor, the United States, in the fight against infectious disease spread.

From the perspective of the United States, old and new infectious diseases present a major danger to the health and welfare of its citizens and to its interests worldwide. By the same token, the control of infectious disease also presents an unparalleled opportunity for U.S. leadership in global public health that could deepen bilateral ties, foster regional cooperation and stability, and burnish the U.S. image globally through the effective exercise of "smart power."[1] As a frontrunner in health and information technology and the largest single contributor to global public health, the United States can both enhance its national and international security and economic interests and demonstrate its commitment to improving human welfare through the promotion of infectious disease control systems abroad. Its record of successful participation in campaigns against infectious disease, such as eradicating smallpox, reinforces its legitimacy in this domain.[2]

Rhetorically, protecting domestic and foreign populations from infectious diseases has become a national priority, and the need to develop foreign capabilities in infectious disease detection and response has received explicit

1. Smart power refers to the ability to obtain what you want through cooptation rather than coercion. Joseph Nye, *Smart Power: The Means to Succeed in World Politics* (New York: Public Affairs, 2005).
2. Ruth Levine, "Healthy Foreign Policy: Bringing Coherence to the Global Health Agenda," in *The White House and the World: A Global Development Agenda for the Next U.S. President*, ed. Nancy Birdsall (Washington, DC: Center for Global Development, 2008), 43–61.

presidential endorsement. In 1996, President Clinton's Decision Directive NSTC-7 "established a national policy to address the threat of emerging infectious diseases through improved domestic and international surveillance, prevention, and response measures."[3] In introducing the new national policy to the public, then vice president Al Gore underscored that the directive instructs the U.S. government, particularly CDC, USAID, and DOD, to work with other nations and international organizations to establish a global infectious disease surveillance and response system, based on regional hubs and linked by modern communications technologies.[4] Shortly after taking office, President Obama announced a new global health initiative that would adopt an integrated approach to fight the spread of infectious diseases while addressing other global health challenges.[5] The president emphasized:

> In the 21st century, disease flows freely across borders and oceans, and, in recent days, the 2009 H1N1 virus has reminded us of the urgent need for action. We cannot wall ourselves off from the world and hope for the best, nor ignore the public health challenges beyond our borders. An outbreak in Indonesia can reach Indiana within days, and public health crises abroad can cause widespread suffering, conflict, and economic contraction. . . . We cannot simply confront individual preventable illnesses in isolation. The world is interconnected, and that demands an integrated approach to global health.[6]

America's military leaders have echoed these sentiments.[7]

In November 2009, the National Security Council document "National Strategy for Countering Biological Threats" reinforced the importance of strengthening foreign capacity in detecting and responding to infectious disease outbreaks, because this capacity is of equal importance in combating naturally occurring or man-made biological threats. President Obama noted that addressing the challenge "requires a comprehensive approach that recognizes the importance of reducing threats from outbreaks of infectious disease whether natural, accidental, or deliberate in nature."[8] Recognizing

---

3.   The White House, "Addressing the Threat of Emerging Infectious Diseases" (Washington, DC: Executive Office of the President, June 12, 1996), www.fas.org/irp/offdocs/pdd_ntsc7.htm.

4.   The White House, "Vice President Announces Policy on Infectious Diseases, New Presidential Policy Calls for Coordinated Approach to Global Issue" (Washington, DC: Executive Office of the President, June 12, 1996), www.fas.org/irp/offdocs/pdd_ntsc7.htm.

5.   The White House, "Statement by the President on Global Health Initiative" (Washington, DC: Executive Office of the President, May 5, 2009), www.whitehouse.gov/the_press_office/Statement-by-the-President-On-Global-Health-Initiative.

6.   Ibid.

7.   Recently, General Anthony C. Zinni and Admiral Leighton W. Smith Jr., retired from the Marine Corps and the Navy respectively, wrote, "Today, our 'enemies' are often conditions—poverty, infectious disease, political instability and corruption, global warming—which generate the biggest threats." "A Smarter Weapon," *USA Today*, March 27, 2008, A11.

8.   The White House, "National Strategy for Countering Biological Threats," presidential directive, letter of transmittal (Washington, DC: Executive Office of the President, November 2009).

growing global interconnectedness, the policy calls for building on bilateral and multilateral partnerships to improve international preparedness by helping countries establish "effective and sustainable systems for disease surveillance, detection, diagnosis, and reporting."[9]

Despite consensus on the importance of the issue and clear recognition that combating the threat of infectious diseases requires support for public health systems abroad, U.S. policies designed to bolster foreign capacity in infectious disease control have not kept pace with America's burgeoning global public health expenditures.

With regard to the finely wrought cooperative regional networks described in chapter 2 and analyzed in chapters 3 and 4 of this book, the U.S. government role has been, and should remain, indirect. For example, U.S. governmental material assistance and training has contributed to the development of substantial epidemiological capacity in Thailand, which in turn is a locus of expertise for the Mekong Basin Disease Surveillance Network. Even though the role of U.S. policy is most appropriately an indirect one of technical assistance and capacity building, this chapter questions whether U.S. policies that indirectly foster regional cooperation and global capacity are enough to meet the challenge to its interests and the opportunity for enhanced cooperation posed by the emergence and potential global spread of old and new infectious diseases. If not, what changes in terms of policies, purse, or bureaucratic organization and coordination might better secure these interests and opportunities?

To explore these questions, this chapter identifies and describes four federal programs designed exclusively to strengthen foreign capacity in infectious disease surveillance and response, considers their interagency and international partnerships, and recommends ways to expand U.S. support for infectious disease control abroad.

U.S. Government Programs

American domestic public health initiatives date to the early years of the republic[10] and the nation's involvement in international public health began in the late 1800s with its participation in the first international sanitary conferences.[11] During and soon after World War II, U.S. military and civilian agencies were often called on to assist in identifying and eradicating disease

---

9.   Ibid., 23.

10.   The origins of America's public health system can be traced to federal legislation of 1798 that established a network of hospitals for the care of merchant seamen.

11.   See chapter 2.

and fortifying international public health systems abroad. Support for overseas public health systems has been part of the mission of the U.S. Agency for International Development (USAID) since its inception in 1961, for example, and the Centers for Disease Control and Prevention (CDC) has been active in the worldwide campaigns to eradicate infectious diseases, such as smallpox, since the 1960s.

Today, U.S. global public health policy is a sprawling and complex enterprise. As of 2008, federal expenditures totaled about $9 billion allocated to eleven executive departments and agencies (plus five multiagency initiatives).[12] The U.S. government has programs in more than 100 countries, and fifteen congressional committees oversee its efforts.[13]

Core support for programs designed exclusively to strengthen international infectious disease surveillance and response, less than $100 million, constitutes about 1 percent of all U.S. government global health expenditures. This figure is inexact, however, because of the way American foreign assistance and global public health policies are characterized and how programs are structured. First, American support for global public health programs are categorized as serving several broad purposes.[14] Because these purposes are complementary, it is not always clear which programs and expenditures fall in which category.[15]

A second and even larger problem for determining the scope of U.S. efforts stems from the vertical rather than horizontal structure of America's global health policies. That is, American programs and funding are directed overwhelmingly toward particular diseases or themes rather than more general objectives such as strengthening overseas infectious disease control systems and coordinating these programs regionally and globally. Initiatives directed at specific diseases such as AIDS, malaria, tuberculosis, and influenza support some activities that improve infectious disease detection and

---

12. The precise figure is impossible to determine because the U.S. government has no agreed definition across agencies of what programs constitute "global health activities." Julie Fisher et al., "U.S. Global Health Policies: Mapping the United States Engagement in Global Public Health" (Menlo Park, CA: Kaiser Family Foundation, August 2009), 1, www.kff.org/globalhealth/upload/7958.pdf.

13. For an excellent overview of the scope of U.S. policy, see Kaiser Family Foundation, "U.S. Global Health Policy, The U.S. Government's Global Health Policy Architecture: Structure Programs, and Funding" (Menlo Park, CA: Kaiser Family Foundation, April 2009), www.kff.org/globalhealth/7881.cfm.

14. These purposes include basic and essential health care services and infrastructure development; disease detection and response, population and maternal/child health, nonemergency nutrition support, clean water/sanitation promotion; and mitigation of environmental hazards. Ibid.

15. For example, programs designed to improve the curriculum and practice in public health management overseas are generally characterized as infrastructure development, not as part of U.S. expenditures on disease detection and response programs. In contrast, programs in support of educational and curriculum development in epidemiology, for instance, are generally considered part of the core expenditures for disease detection and response. The delineation is somewhat imprecise, if not arbitrary.

response abroad through interagency funds transferred to programs that pursue this mission, and indirectly to the extent that their programs have system strengthening dimension. The amount of related interagency transfers varies from program to program and from one year to the next, as do the funds secured from private donors that augment U.S. infectious disease control programs abroad.

Given these caveats, this chapter focuses on four programs shared by three federal departments that are explicitly aimed at improving the infectious disease detection and response capabilities of other nations and regions:[16]

- the Global Disease Detection Program operated by the CDC, which is part of the Department of Health and Human Services (HHS);
- the Field Epidemiology and Laboratory Training Program administered by the CDC with significant support from USAID;[17]
- the Integrated Disease Surveillance and Response Program funded primarily by USAID and administered through CDC; and
- the Global Emerging Infections Surveillance and Response System of the U.S. Department of Defense.

In addition to these four programs, USAID provides bilateral in-country support to public health programs in most of the more than 100 countries in which it operates, estimated at $14 million in 2006.[18]

These four programs, like U.S. support for global health programs generally, have long pedigrees. Each of the three federal departments or agencies directly responsible for infectious disease surveillance and response has supported foreign capacity building for many years. Within the last decade, however, these four programs have emerged as distinct policy initiatives.

Global Disease Detection Program

In 2004, shortly after the SARS epidemic, Congress appropriated funds for CDC to create the Global Disease Detection (GDD) program. Recognizing that a weakness in the infectious disease surveillance system of any country

---

16. This approach is consistent with the scope of investigation adopted by the General Accountability Office (GAO) in its report, "Global Health: U.S. Agencies Support Programs to Build Overseas Capacity for Infectious Disease Surveillance," statement by David Gootnik, director of International Affairs and Trade, GAO-08-138T (Washington, DC: Government Printing Office, October 4, 2007), www.gao.gov/new.items/d08138t.pdf.
17. USAID is technically an independent agency of the federal government, but works under the policy direction of the Department of State, which has statutory authority over its budget.
18. GAO, "Global Health," 7.

potentially imperils U.S. and global interests, Congress directed the program to "protect the health of Americans and the global community by developing and strengthening public health capacity to rapidly detect and respond to emerging infectious diseases and bioterrorist threats."[19] The program draws on CDC's long-standing expertise in infectious disease detection and response to support overseas public health surveillance, provide training and laboratory methods, build in-country capacity, and enhance rapid response for emerging infectious diseases.

CDC has established six GDD centers—one in each WHO region—to serve the needs of that country and neighboring states: Thailand (2004), Kenya (2004), Guatemala (2006), Egypt (2006), China (2006), and Kazakhstan (2008). Start-up activities at a seventh GDD regional center are under way. CDC has aspirations to eventually establish eighteen centers worldwide as regional resources to detect, confirm, and respond to pathogens at the source. Consistent with the goals of IHR 2005,[20] GDD helps host countries develop core capacities in six areas: emerging infectious disease detection and response, training in field epidemiology and laboratory methods, pandemic influenza preparedness and response, zoonotic disease investigation, health communication and information technology, and laboratory systems and biosafety.

Funding for the program grew rapidly from $11.6 million at its inception in fiscal year (FY) 2004, to $32.4 million in FY 2006 and held relatively steady at $31.4 million in FY 2008 and $33.7 million in 2009.[21] Fiscal year appropriations for 2010 were $37.8 million and remained the same in the 2011 budget request. Staffing for the program includes 33 employees based overseas, 649 locally employed staff overseas, and an oversight team of 30 employees based in CDC's Atlanta headquarters.[22]

CDC qualitatively and quantitatively monitors the outputs, outcomes, and, where possible, the overall impact, of the GDD programs with respect to the five key capacities: outbreak response, surveillance, pathogen discovery, training, and networking. In 2009, CDC reported that during the period

---

19. CDC, "Global Disease Detection Policy Paper" (Atlanta, GA: Centers for Disease Control and Prevention, June 2008), www.cdc.gov/cogh/pdf/GDD_at_a_Glance_2008.pdf.

20. Article 44 of the IHR directs state parties to collaborate with each other to detect, assess, and respond to events and to develop, strengthen, and maintain public health capacities.

21. GDD program expenditures averaged 6.8 percent of CDC's annual global health expenditures during this period. Tiaji Salaam-Blyther, "Centers for Disease Control and Prevention Global Health Programs: FY2001–FY2010" (Washington, DC: Congressional Research Service, August 2009), http://fpc.state.gov/documents/organization/128822.pdf.

22. CDC, "Global Disease and Detection Program: Monitoring and Evaluation Report 2006–2008" (Atlanta, GA: Centers for Disease Control and Prevention, June 2009), 4, www.cdc.gov/globalhealth/GDD/pdf/GDD_m&e.pdf.

from 2006 through year-end 2009 it had achieved the following capacity-building metrics:

Outbreak response—provided rapid response to more than 500 disease outbreaks and other serious public health emergencies, including Rift Valley fever in Kenya, cholera in Thailand, dengue hemorrhagic fever in Guatemala, anthrax in Kazakhstan, and human influenza A (H5N1) (bird flu) in Egypt. The GDD program also claims to have built national and regional capacity to ensure that outbreak response are demonstrably faster and more reliable resulting in lives saved.

Pathogen discovery—detected thirty-four new pathogens and increased the overall number of pathogens identified locally from eleven in 2006 to sixty-nine in 2009. This growing base of knowledge facilitates early identification of outbreaks and appropriate response interventions.

Training—increased the number of Field Epidemiology Training Program (FETP) graduates working in the GDD Centers from 26 in 2006 to 160 in 2008. Short-term public health training was provided to more than thirty-seven thousand participants worldwide.

Surveillance—all six GDD centers are conducting surveillance systems or projects with the goal of making policy recommendations, evaluating interventions, and measuring the public health impact of new initiatives.

Networking—WHO use of the GDD network as part of the international response to the 2009 outbreak of novel influenza A (H1N1) (swine flu).[23]

CDC coordinates the work of the GDD centers with the WHO, particularly its regional offices for the Americas, the Pan American Health Organization (PAHO), and the Regional Office for Africa (AFRO). GDD Regional Centers also function as members of the WHO's Global Outbreak Alert and Response Network (GOARN) during emergencies. The GDD program collaborates and supports the work of numerous NGOs and philanthropies working in this policy space. CDC's Center for Global Health at its Atlanta headquarters oversees these and other partnerships.[24]

Field Epidemiology and Laboratory Training Program

The CDC's Field Epidemiology Training Program (FETP) and the Field Epidemiological and Laboratory Training Program (FELTP) are applied

---

23. For a qualitative and quantitative assessment, see CDC, "Global Disease Detection Program: Monitoring and Evaluation Report 2006–2008." See also CDC, "Global Disease Detection Program, Fact Sheet: GDD Accomplishments" (Atlanta, GA: Centers for Disease Control and Prevention, 2009), www.cdc.gov/globalhealth/GCC/accomplishments_2006-Q1and2-2009.pdf.

24. CDC, "Coordinating Office for Global Health," www.cdc.gov/cogh/partnership.html.

epidemiology education programs designed to help foreign countries, develop, run, and sustain a robust public health infrastructure. The programs are established in cooperation with ministries of health around the world and in concert with national and international partners.[25] The goal is both to build up host country epidemiological and laboratory capacity and thereby contribute to evidence-based public health decision making that will improve the host country's overall health and safety policies.

Started in 1980, the programs provide two years of applied training for public health leaders to strengthen disease surveillance and assessment skills and to improve health interventions. The FELTP program, as the name implies, includes a laboratory-training component, is modeled after CDC's domestic Epidemic Intelligence Service, and is adapted to meet the particular needs of the host country. Before initiating a program, the CDC requires a serious commitment from the recipient country, including material support, and expects that the recipient country will own the program and that eventually the program will become fully self-sustaining. Planning for the creation of a FE(L)TP program typically takes up to two years to ensure its initial success and guarantee its long-term adoption and sustainability by the host nation. As one official explained, "we go into the project with an exit strategy."[26] The costs to set up a FE(L)TP program is estimated to be in the range of $1 to $2 million, primarily to support an in-country resident advisor and training and materials.

FELTP and FETP trainees typically take courses in epidemiology, communication, economics, management, and methodology. They spend the majority of their time in the field conducting epidemiological investigation and surveys, evaluating surveillance systems and prevention practices, and training other health workers. A team of CDC professionals develops and delivers most of the curriculum and CDC assigns an in-country advisor for four to six years to provide training and technical assistance.[27] Directorship of the program remains the responsibility of the host nation, however.

Over the course of the program, CDC has consulted with and supported thirty-one programs involving forty countries that have produced more than 1,500 graduates. CDC has established nineteen previously funded,

25. CDC, "Global Health: Field Epidemiology Training Program," www.cdc.gov/globalhealth/FETP.

26. Personal interview, Atlanta, GA, January 29, 2010.

27. CDC, "Division of Global Public Health Capacity Development, 2008 Annual Report" (Atlanta, GA: Centers for Disease Control and Prevention, 2009), www.cdc.gov/globalhealth/FETP/pdf/2008_annual_report_508.pdf.

self-sustaining FETP programs.[28] As of 2010, CDC had eighteen resident advisors supporting twelve ongoing programs involving twenty-three countries.[29] Twelve programs engaging seventeen countries are in various stages of development.[30]

In addition to the continuation of country programs and their eventual graduation to self-sustainability, there are other measures of long-term impact. A 2007 internal analysis of six FETP programs established between 1999 and 2004, for example, revealed that 92 percent of the graduates continued to work in public health after graduation.[31] With regard to program assessment, CDC has developed and is piloting a self-administered scorecard for FE(L)TP programs to measure progress regarding the quality and sustainability of their programs.[32] Assigning responsibility for assessment and improvement of the program to the host country with CDC and other international partners playing a supporting role is consistent with the programs emphasis on self-reliance.

In conducting its work, the CDC regularly collaborates with international organizations, particularly the World Health Organization and World Bank; other U.S. agencies and departments such as USAID, State, and Defense; and private actors such as the Gates Foundation, Ellison Medical Foundation, the Rockefeller Foundation, and the Carter Center.[33] Core CDC budget for the program has been roughly steady since 2005 at approximately $3 million per year.[34] By leveraging its resources with transfers from other federal agencies and programs, particularly from USAID and private donors, total program expenditures in fiscal year 2010 approached $25 million.[35] The

28. In order of date established, these include programs in Thailand, Mexico, Taiwan, Saudi Arabia, Philippines, Peru, Australia, Colombia, Italy, Egypt, Zimbabwe, Span, Uganda, Germany, Vietnam, Japan, Brazil, and India. CDC, "2010 Field Epidemiology and Management Capacity Building Programs" (unpublished internal document).

29. These include Central America (Costa Rica, Dominican Republic, El Salvador, Guatemala, and Honduras); Central Asia (Kazakhstan, Kyrgyzstan, Tajikistan, Turkmenistan, and Uzbekistan); China, Ethiopia, Ghana, India (Chennai and New Delhi); Kenya (including South Sudan); Nigeria; Pakistan; South Africa; the South Caucasus (Armenia, Azerbaijan, and Georgia); and, Tanzania. CDC, "2010 Field Epidemiology and Management."

30. Countries with programs under development include Afghanistan, Angola, Bangladesh, Belize, Central Africa (Cameroon, Central African Republic, and Democratic Republic of Congo), Iraq, Morocco, Mozambique, Panama, Paraguay, Rwanda, and West Africa (Burkina Faso, Mali, Niger, and Togo). CDC, "2010 Field Epidemiology and Management" (unpublished internal document, January 2010).

31. The six programs examined were those in Brazil, Central Asia, Central America, India, Jordan, and Kenya. GAO, "Global Health: U.S. Agencies Support Programs to Build Overseas Capacity for Infectious Disease Surveillance."

32. CDC, "Capacity Development News," Spring 2009, www.cdc.gov/globalhealth/FETP/pdf/2009_newsletter_508.pdf.

33. CDC, "Division of Global Public Health Capacity Development 2008 Annual Report."

34. GAO, "Global Health."

35. Personal interview, Atlanta, GA, January 29, 2010.

Center for Global Health also has administrative coordination responsibility for the FELP and FELTP programs through the Division of Global Public Health Capacity Building.

Countries that set up FE(L)TP programs can collaborate with two field epidemiology nonprofit network organizations to share resources and best practices. The two organizations are the international Training Programs in Epidemiology and Public Health Interventions Network (TEPHI-NET) and the regional African Field Epidemiology Network (AFENET). TEPHINET, which is headquartered in Atlanta, was incorporated in 1999 as a nonprofit organization with the aim of strengthening international public health capacity through the support and networking of field-based training programs that enhance competencies in applied epidemiology and public health practice. Approximately forty country programs participate in TEPHINET today. TEPHINET receives support from the CDC, USAID, WHO, and the Gates and Google Foundations. Created in 2005, AFENET is a nonprofit voluntary alliance dedicated to helping ministries of health in Africa build strong, effective, sustainable health systems through FETP and FELTP programs and for the sharing of regional expertise in field epidemiology and laboratory practice. Headquartered in Kampala, Uganda, the organization has seven full members, eight associate members, and six potential members.[36] Financial supporters and partners to AFENET include CDC, USAID, WHO, private foundations, and university medical schools.

Integrated Disease Surveillance and Response Program

Integrated Disease Surveillance and Response (IDSR) is a strategy of the World Health Organization African Regional Office (WHO-AFRO) adopted by member states in 1998 and supported by the CDC. The IDSR strategy focuses on developing surveillance systems, monitoring and evaluating those systems, and strengthening laboratory capabilities and workforce training. The emphasis is on a multilevel, multidisease[37] surveillance and response system that could integrate activities from the district, state, and provincial level to the national level. The integrated approach strives to

---

36. Full members include Ghana, Kenya, Nigeria, South Africa, Tanzania, Uganda, and Zimbabwe. Associate members include: Ethiopia, Rwanda, South Sudan, Burkina Faso, Mali, Niger, and Togo. Potential members include: Angola, Cameroon, the Central African Republic, the Democratic Republic of Congo, and Mozambique. See AFENET, wwwafenet.net/english/about.php.

37. The IDSR strategy targeted nineteen priority communicable diseases divided into three categories: epidemic-prone diseases, diseases targeted for eradication and elimination, and diseases that are endemic. A directive from WHO-AFRO added pandemic influenza to the IDSR list. Helen N. Perry et al., "Planning an Integrated Disease Surveillance and Response System: A Matrix of Skills and Activities," *BMC Medicine* 5 (2007): 24–32, doi:10.1186/1741-7015-5-24.

develop and maximize the potential of a resource-constrained country to promote public health, increase flexibility to respond to emerging threats, and meet the international standards for disease reporting and control set by the WHO in its IHR 2005.[38]

CDC has provided technical assistance to the IDSR program since its inception through WHO-AFRO and various African ministries of health in a broad effort that involves three CDC divisions.[39] CDC provides expertise in the design, development, implementation, monitoring, and evaluation of IDSR strategies and tools for disease surveillance and laboratory confirmation.[40] CDC considers laboratory support and networking of labs for information sharing across the public health infrastructure to be especially important to a country's public health surveillance system.[41] The CDC annual budget for the program is about $3 million. The work of the IDSR system is designed to complement other related efforts such as the FE(L)TP program by coordinating and streamlining surveillance activities so as to maximize available resources like epidemiological and lab skills developed by FE(L)TP.

A participating country begins the implementation of IDSR with an assessment of the national surveillance system using a team of national and international experts to examine the current surveillance, laboratory confirmation, and epidemic preparedness and response activities at all levels of a country's health system. The ministry of health then uses the assessment results to develop a plan of action for creating a fully functional IDSR system including improvements at the national, provincial, district, health facility, and community levels of the health system. In its early years, WHO-AFRO focused primarily on strengthening capacity and coordination at the district level. The first implementation activity is the adaptation of the WHO generic surveillance and response tools to reflect national policies.[42]

The IDSR network grew rapidly from 2001 to 2005, the number of countries with a developed IDSR plan of action increasing from thirteen in 2001

---

38. Ibid.
39. The divisions include: the Division of Emerging Infections and Surveillance Services (DEISS), the Division of Epidemiology and Surveillance Capacity Development (DESCD), and the Global Immunization Division (GID), National Immunization Program. These three divisions share funding, materials, and resources for IDSR activities and engage experts in other CDC programs and public health agencies as needed.
40. CDC, "Division of Emerging Infections and Surveillance Services (DEISS)," www.cdc.gov/ncpdcid/deiss/index.html.
41. Jean-Bosco Ndihokubwayo et al., "Guide for National Public Health Laboratory Networking to Strengthen Integrated Disease Surveillance and Response" (WHO-AFRO and CDC unpublished internal report, test version 1.0, September 2008).
42. CDC, "Integrated Disease Surveillance and Response," www.cdc.gov/idsr/about.

to forty-one in 2005 and those with an established national IDSR committee expanding from six to thirty-two in the same time frame.[43] Since that time, the program has slowed to allow for the incorporation of the new requirements mandated by IHR 2005 into the IDSR programs and owing to a turnover in personnel at several national and regional WHO-AFRO offices.

The countries themselves are largely responsible for conducting assessment of the program. A WHO-AFRO task force, with input from the CDC and USAID, adopted IDSR core indicators in 2003. Participating countries use the IDSR core indicators to monitor and evaluate their progress to ensure that they maintain effective and functional IDSR systems. Countries also use the results to identify problems and make corrections to improve the quality of the surveillance information and the overall performance of the system.[44] U.S. agencies cannot require countries to collect data on these indicators, however, because IDSR is a country-owned program. In 2006, nineteen of the forty-six participating countries reported on at least some of the indicators. In 2005, the CDC completed an evaluation of IDSR implementation progress in Ghana, Tanzania, Uganda and Zimbabwe, finding that these countries had implemented most of the ISDR framework. In addition, WHO-AFRO conducts periodic in-depth assessments of country progress.[45]

Partner countries and their international partners work together on strategies and activities toward common goals for the WHO African region, sharing their experiences and achievements and setting goals for the upcoming year. A biannual newsletter on IDSR progress and plans has also been published and a monthly bulletin, the *Communicable Diseases Epidemiological Report*, provides updates of IDSR activities and progress, and reports of surveillance data of priority infectious diseases in the African region.[46]

Global Emerging Infections Surveillance and Response System

Historically, infectious disease has had a direct negative effect on military forces and operations by its debilitating effects. Today, the U.S. Department of Defense has personnel deployed to at least 147 countries around the world, and has a presence of more than 200 personnel in at least twenty-one

---

43. Ibid.
44. Ibid.
45. See, for example, Luswa Lukwago et al., "The Implementation of Integrated Disease Surveillance and Response in Uganda: A Review of Progress and Challenges between 2001 and 2007" (unpublished internal document, Kampala: Ministry of Health Uganda and WHO Uganda Country Office).
46. CDC, "Integrated Disease Surveillance and Response Partners," www.cdc.gov/idsr/partners.htm.

nations.[47] Given this widespread dispersion of military forces, DOD has long maintained systems designed to detect and respond to infectious diseases to maintain force readiness and to protect its employees. The DOD, like some civilian agencies, has a separate and sizable account to support its influenza surveillance, diagnostic, and response activities and, in all, more than a dozen DOD entities and their foreign military partners work together on infectious disease detection and control.[48]

Intersecting many of these programs and integrating overseas research laboratories and humanitarian assistance programs is the Global Emerging Infections Surveillance and Response System (GEIS). DOD created GEIS in response to President Clinton's Decision Directive NSTC-7, "to strengthen the prevention of, surveillance of, and response to infectious disease that (1) are a threat to military personnel and families, (2) reduce medical readiness, or (3) present a risk to U.S. security."[49] GEIS increasingly interprets this mandate broadly to include encouragement of host country capacities in infectious disease control capability and that country's compliance with the IHR 2005. President Obama's National Strategy for Countering Biological Threats further emphasizes the national security threat posed by a man-made or naturally occurring biological outbreak.[50]

GEIS works with various research and treatment facilities operated by DOD to improve their ability to provide early detection of emerging infectious disease threats, to facilitate information sharing in disease surveillance and research, and to enhance response capabilities with a particular focus on five categories of infectious diseases: respiratory disease (particularly influenza), gastroenteritis syndromes, febrile illnesses (such as dengue fever and malaria), antimicrobial resistance (a particular problem in tuberculosis), and sexually transmitted infections.[51]

---

47. Lawrence Kapp and Don J. Jansen, "The Role of the Department of Defense during a Flu Pandemic," Congressional Research Service Report, June 2009, www.fas.org/sgp/crs/natsec/R40619.pdf, 3–4.

48. Congress passed legislation in 1986 that extended the permissible scope of DOD's humanitarian assistance programs to include noncrisis projects that provided health services in the context of overall military operations. This legislation enabled the creation of various military-to-military collaborations in health capacity building and joint research projects in developing nations. Julie Fisher et al., "U.S. Global Health Policies: Mapping the United States Engagement in Global Public Health" (Menlo Park, CA: Kaiser Family Foundation, August 2009), 23.

49. Eugene V. Bonventre, Kathleen H. Hicks, and Stacy M Okutani, "U.S. National Security and Global Health: An Analysis of Global Health Engagement by the U.S. Department of Defense" (Washington, DC: Center for Strategic and International Studies, April 2009), http://csis.org/files/publication/090421_Bonventre_USNationalSecurity_Rev.pdf.

50. White House, "National Strategy for Countering Biological Threats," November 2009.

51. DOD, Global Emerging Infections Surveillance and Response System, "Fiscal Year 2008 Annual Report," http://afhsc.mil/viewDocument?file=GEIS/GEISAnnRpt08.pdf, 6.

In FY 2009, DOD obligated approximately $12 million to core surveillance capacity building for GEIS, up from $8 million in 2005.[52] Separately, GEIS received $40 million in supplemental funds as part of the government's efforts targeted on pandemic and avian influenza. These funds help support research laboratories in Egypt, Indonesia, Kenya, Peru, and Thailand as well as other military research units for surveillance projects located in seventy-eight countries.[53] Many of these projects are conducted with host country nationals, often in the form of military-to-military cooperation, and include establishing or enhancing laboratories, training host country staff in surveillance techniques, and providing advanced diagnostic equipment.[54] The labs themselves remain DOD assets and belong to particular branches of the armed services.

In February 2008, GEIS became a core component of the newly formed Armed Forces Health Surveillance Center (AFHSC).[55] Within this new organizational framework, the GEIS continues to promote and facilitate national and international preparedness for emerging infections while maintaining its focus on protecting the health of all DOD health care beneficiaries. GEIS's mission statement for "2009 and beyond" includes the following four goals: surveillance and response; training and capacity building; research, innovation, and integration; and assessment and communication of value added.[56]

No formal overall monitoring and evaluation framework is in place for GEIS, though assessment and reporting on particular programs is undertaken quarterly and annually. As in civilian programs, developing metrics for overall effectiveness and impact is difficult in this area. Success in terms of disease prevention is hard to quantify and country baselines against which to measure performance can be difficult to obtain.[57]

Regarding interagency coordination, a 2007 GAO study gave the program solid marks for its efforts at interagency communication,[58] but a GEIS

---

52. Before 2005, GEIS was not a separately tallied budget item. Rather its support was included in the various laboratories it supported.

53. DOD, "Fiscal Year 2008 Annual Report." In addition to research conducted in overseas laboratories, each branch of the military services maintains U.S.-based research programs and laboratories that focus on infectious diseases in addition to other medical issues such as occupational and environmental health. Kaiser Family Foundation, "U.S. Global Health," 14.

54. GAO, "Global Health," 3.

55. Now known as the GEIS Operations Division of the AFHSC, GEIS joins the Defense Medical Surveillance System and the DOD Serum Repository as part of a larger and more diverse organization serving the DOD.

56. DOD, "Fiscal Year 2008 Annual Report."

57. Personal interview, Washington, DC, March 2, 2010.

58. GAO, "Global Health."

annual report concedes that coordination and collaboration with its inter-agency and international partners such as the WHO remains challenging because the organizations are immense bureaucracies with constantly chang-ing personnel. A 2008 study by the independent Institute of Medicine encouraged GEIS to enhance its coordination and collaboration with its domestic counterparts, particularly the CDC, which operates in almost all the countries that have DOD laboratories.[59]

Assessment of U.S. Policy

As far as they go, there is little wrong and much right about U.S. programs in support of improving foreign capacity in infectious disease surveillance and response. The problem is that they do not go far enough. The failure to ad-equately engage the threat of infectious disease outbreaks at the source and to seize the potential opportunity for enduring international collaborations in public health is both a security lapse and a foregone opportunity for the effective exercise of American influence.

This shortcoming reflects generic problems in U.S. global health policies, including several tendencies of American global health policy:

- to fund treatment for a few diseases rather than strengthen public health systems generally to enable them to respond to existing and emerging challenges;
- to focus overwhelmingly on treating the problem of infectious disease spread only after it has reached U.S. shores;
- to offer charity rather than make investments in host countries;
- to deploy funding in response to the current interests of the donor community and to focus on near-term impact rather than concentrate on recipient needs and sustainable, long-run effects; and
- to support related programs in various agencies without a formal mechanism for interagency coordination and collaboration.

Are programmatic funding levels enough to meet the threat of infectious disease spread and the promise of improved diplomatic relations through strengthening overseas capacity in disease control? The short answer is no. This conclusion comes despite the fact that U.S. support of global public health has expanded rapidly in the past decade. During that period, U.S. funding for global health programs has quintupled from $1.7 billion in FY

---

59. IOM, *Review of the DOD-GEIS Influenza Programs* (Washington, DC: National Academies Press, 2008), 12.

Figure 5. Funding for U.S. Global Health Programs FY 2004–10

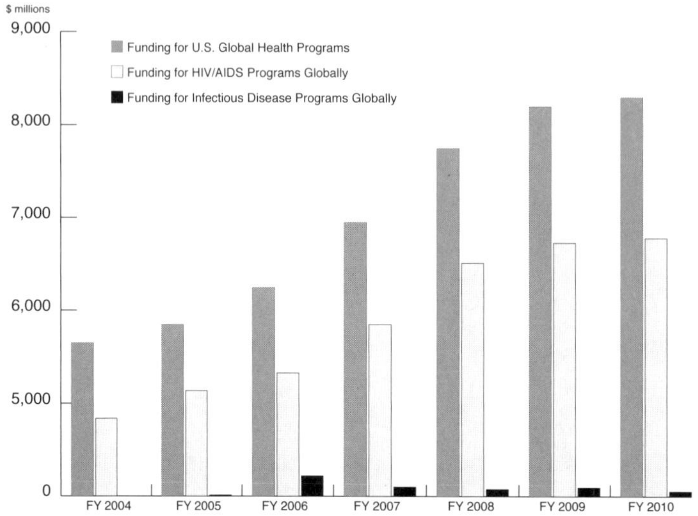

$ millions

- ■ Funding for U.S. Global Health Programs
- ☐ Funding for HIV/AIDS Programs Globally
- ■ Funding for Infectious Disease Programs Globally

Source: Jen Kates, "The U.S. Global Health Initiative Overview and Budget Analysis," Kaiser Family Foundation, December 2009.

2001 to $8.8 billion in FY 2010. The president's FY 2011 budget request anticipates another increase in funding to $9.6 billion.[60]

Notwithstanding the growing pie, funding for long-term programs that strengthen global capacity in infectious disease surveillance and response remains small and relatively stagnant, especially for civilian programs, as seen in figure 5.

A decade ago, the GAO, an independent assessment body of the U.S. government, noted the need to do more to strengthen overseas laboratory capacity, improve disease surveillance, and prevent the spread of diseases in developing countries through greater support of programs like the GDD and the FE(L)TP.[61] Nonetheless, core budgets for these programs have not increased in real terms since 2006.[62]

The status of the GDD program illustrates the implications of under funding. As noted, the GDD aspires to create eighteen linked regional and subregional centers for infectious disease control around the world—a network first called for in President Clinton's 1996 directive. To date,

60. Jen Kates, "The U.S. Global Health Initiative: Overview and Budget Analysis," Kaiser Family Foundation, December 2009, http://kff.org/globalhealth/upload/8009.pdf. The increases in U.S. support parallel increases in global assistance for public health. See Nirmala Ravishshankar et al., "Financing Global Health: Tracking Development Assistance for Health from 1990 to 2007," *The Lancet* 373 (June 20, 2009): 2113–24.

61.   GAO, "Challenges in Improving Infectious Disease Surveillance Systems," GAO-01-722 (Washington, DC: Government Printing Office, August 2001), 35, www.goa.gov/new.items/d01722.pdf.

62.   See Salaam-Blyther, "Centers for Disease Control."

Figure 6. GDD Growth Matrix

	Emerging Infections	Field Epidemiology	Influenza	Zoonoses	Health Community and IT	Lab Systems and Biosafety
Thailand						
Kenya						
Guatemala						
China						
Egypt						
Kazahkstan						
India	FY2009	FY2009				
Bangladesh						
Mexico						
Brazil						
South Africa						
West Africa						
TBD: Using risk-based approach						18 GDD Centers

Increased Capacity

Increased Coverage

Current capability   Partial capability   * Potential location for placement of a GDD regional center

Source: Center for Global Health, Division of Global Disease Detection and Emergency Response, CDC, March 5, 2010

however, that network is not in place; only six centers are completed and a seventh is in progress. To fully implement the program, GDD's budget would need to increase approximately six-fold to about $200 million. The U.S. government should not wait until an infectious disease disaster occurs to begin filling in the gaps in this system. Figure 6 shows the many gaps remaining in the program.

In the context of U.S. global health expenditures generally, the core budgets of programs designed to strengthen overseas capacity in infectious disease surveillance and response are very small. Rather than increasing core budgets to meet a critical, long-term need, the primary agencies and programs have authority to seek funds from disease-specific programs through interagency transfers or to secure donations from international organizations or private philanthropies to meet their programmatic objectives. Although these governmental programs have been effective and entrepreneurial in augmenting their budgets, such an ad hoc, opportunistic funding model does not allow for systematic planning and expansion of programs to meet a stated national priority.

As described, U.S. spending for global public health has ballooned in recent years, but the increase in funding has gone overwhelmingly to fighting a handful of diseases and in particular to treating HIV/AIDS. Since the launch of the President's Emergency Plan for AIDS Relief (PEPFAR) in 2003, more than 70 percent of U.S. global health funds have been allocated to AIDS programs.[63] The proposed 2011 budget would continue this trend, with nearly $7 billion of the proposed $9.6 billion going to PEPFAR.[64] Not only does an overwhelming percentage of U.S. funding go toward treating one disease, during the first five years and $15 billion of the PEPFAR initiative, funds were earmarked for treatment largely in the form of antiretroviral drugs (55 percent), palliative care (20 percent), prevention (20 percent), and care of HIV/AIDS orphans and vulnerable populations (10 percent)—leaving little to fund efforts designed to strengthen public health capacity in recipient countries.[65]

The PEPFAR initiative has been a powerful impetus for garnering support for global health programs generally, and is remarkable for its generosity and the number of lives it has saved and enhanced. Focusing on treating one disease, however, leaves other health problems unattended and limits capacity building in core areas such as epidemiology and laboratory capability.[66] Capacity building is critical to combating infectious disease generally and to making the entire health system robust and grounded in sound science and reliable data. PEPFAR's own analysis of its first five years concludes that the program has largely ignored the issue of strategic strengthening of health systems in the countries in which it operates, has "had both positive and negative impacts on country-level health systems," and that programs "did not fully translate to a broader service delivery impact across the health sector."[67] The consequence, health analyst Julie Fisher concludes, is that "U.S. support for disease-specific programs [saves] lives but leaves most of the population without essential services, does little to free human capital for economic development, or to accomplish either public health or soft diplomacy goals."[68] Other disease specific programs that have grown more gradually have had a greater opportunity to balance short-run treatment with

---

63. National Academies, "Global Health Should Be a Key Component of U.S. Foreign Policy," press release, December 15, 2008, www8.nationalacademies.org/opinews/newsitem.aspx?.

64. This amount includes $1 billion committed through the Global Fund.

65. Levine, "Healthy Foreign Policy," 49.

66. On this problem, see, for example, Colleen C. Denny and Ezekial J. Emanuel, "U.S. Health Aid Beyond PEPFAR: The Mother and Child Campaign," *JAMA* 300, no. 17 (November 5, 2008): 2048–15; Eduardo Gomez, "Stop Fighting Viruses, Start Treating People," *Foreign Policy*, January 27, 2010, www.foreignpolicy.com/articles/2010/01/27/stop_fighting_viruses_start_treating_people?page=0,1; Colin D. Mathers and Dejan Loncar, "Projections of Global Mortality and Burden of Disease for 2002 to 2030," *PLOS Medicine* 3, no. 11 (2006): 2111–30.

67. Department of State, "The U.S. President's Emergency Plan for AIDS Relief: Five-Year Strategy" (Washington DC, December 2009), 8, 12, www.pepfar.gov/strategy/document/index.htm.

68. Julie E. Fischer, "Silos within Silos: Unknotting U.S. Global Health Initiatives," December 15, 2009, http://budgetinsight.wordpress.com/2009/12/15/silos-within-silos-unknotting-u-s-global-health-initiatives/.

Figure 7. Infectious Disease Deaths by Region, 2004

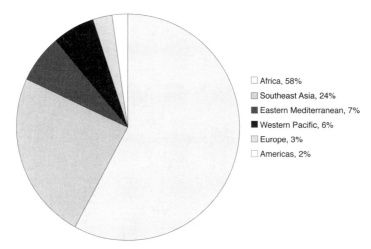

☐ Africa, 58%
▨ Southeast Asia, 24%
■ Eastern Mediterranean, 7%
■ Western Pacific, 6%
▨ Europe, 3%
☐ Americas, 2%

Source: WHO, *Global Burden of Disease 2004,* 54–55. http://whqlibdoc.who.int/publications/2008/9789241563710_eng.pdf.

long-run system building and sustainability and, in time, this may prove true of PEPFAR too.[69]

U.S. disease-specific support in the case of pandemic influenza, illustrates a second problem with the focus of U.S. funding: the tendency to spend funds overwhelmingly on domestic preparedness, rather than creating a front line of defense by detecting and controlling infectious disease outbreaks at the source, that is to say primarily in Africa and Asia as reflected in figure 7.[70]

When the United States responded to the swine flu outbreak with a supplemental appropriation of more than $6.5 billion in 2009, for example, only $190 million of that amount went to global programs, the balance spent largely on domestic defensive countermeasures.[71] Of course, domestic programs such a vaccine stockpiling are essential to protect Americans, but the issue is whether an ounce of protection achieved by putting a higher priority on global overseas surveillance and response capacity is worth a pound of domestic medical cure. In considering that question, a recent study by the Center for Strategic and International Studies concluded that efforts to support overseas capacity in infectious disease surveillance and response "will

---

69. Personal interview, Washington, DC, March 9, 2010.
70. Levine, "Healthy Foreign Policy," 46.
71. Sarah A. Lister, and C. Stephen Redhead, "The 2009 Influenza Pandemic: An Overview" (Washington, DC: Congressional Research Service, September 10, 2009), http://assets.opencrs.com/rpts/R40554_20090910.pdf.

likely benefit U.S. national security more than U.S.-based countermeasure efforts have to date, while also working to improve health during times of peace."[72] Long-term investments in support of surveillance programs overseas is an efficient way to support resource-poor countries as they develop their national surveillance and overall public health infrastructure and to enhance transnational capacity for disease control.[73]

The failure to strengthen foreign capacity reflects a U.S. tendency to give money for treatment of particular diseases rather than invest for the long-term in public health infrastructure abroad.[74] This approach persists despite the fact that viable health systems are key to curtailing the spread of infectious disease and improving the overall health of the recipient country.[75]

Investment in foreign public health capacity is limited for several reasons, but not particularly sound policy ones. First, demonstrating to appropriators and their constituents the direct, quantifiable impact of bolstering overseas public health systems is difficult. Lives not lost to disease, infections prevented by early detection, and pandemics avoided by rapid containment at the source are not as easily calculated or as compelling as immediate, measurable effects of a program that vaccinates or treats thousands or millions of patients for a particular illness. Second, system strengthening takes time to realize and appreciate. One analyst recommends a time frame of ten to fifteen years for measuring systemic health impacts.[76] Policymakers in donor countries rarely think in terms beyond the current budget or electoral cycle, however, and are unlikely to make such patient investments. Third, because funding for global health primarily reflects the popular interests of the donor country (the United States) rather than the needs of the recipient country, American expenditures do not always align with the recipient's national health plans or support the recipient's overall public health and treatment infrastructures so as to maximize long-run returns on foreign investment through a true partnership

---

72. Harley Feldbaum, "U.S. Global Health and Security Policy" (Washington, DC: Center for Strategic and International Studies Global Health Policy Center, April 2009), 11, http://csis.org/files/media/csis/pubs/090420_feldbaum_usglobalhealth.pdf.

73. Ann Marie Kimball et al., "Regional Infectious Disease Surveillance Networks and Their Potential to Facilitate the Implementation of the International Health Regulations," *Medical Clinics North America* 92 (2008): 1468.

74. Laurie Garrett and Kammerle Schneider, "Global Health: Getting It Right," in *Health and Development*, eds. Anna Gati and Andrea Boggio (New York: Palgrave Macmillan, 2009), 11.

75. The WHO states that a functioning health system should include access to a well-performing health workforce; essential medical products, vaccines, and technologies; adequate financing; and strategic policy frameworks to provide effective analysis, oversight, and governance. See IOM, "The U.S. Commitment to Global Health: Recommendations for the New Administration" (Washington, DC: National Academies Press, 2009), 14.

76. Levine, "Healthy Foreign Policy," 47.

between donor and recipient. Finally, despite rhetoric to the contrary, U.S. policy still reflects too little appreciation of global interconnectedness and that U.S. interests defined in security, welfare, diplomatic, and humanitarian terms require significant investment abroad as well as at home. When it comes to sustained support of foreign capacity in infectious disease surveillance and response, our investment shortfall leaves the United States and its global interests unnecessarily vulnerable and the country's positive diplomatic influence insufficiently realized.

The Obama administration has heard these critiques and its early policy planning—as reflected in PEPFAR's second five-year strategy document and the President's Global Health Initiative Consultative Document—appears responsive. For example, in its second five-year cycle, PEPFAR aims to "focus on transitioning from an emergency response to promoting sustainable country programs," that serve a broader health and development context, including, for example, training and retaining health care workers critical to all functions of a health care system.[77] Similarly, GHI sets out a broader set of global health priorities. Rather than focusing on particular diseases, the GHI emphasizes upgrading the health care systems and infrastructure of recipient countries. The vision statement for the president's policy explains that "the GHI will help partner countries improve health outcomes through strengthened health systems with a particular focus on improving the health of women, newborns, and children through programs including infectious disease, nutrition, maternal and child health, and safe water." The GHI recognizes that "building functioning systems will, in some cases, require a new way of thinking about health investments, with increased attention to the appropriate deployment of health professionals, improved distribution of medical supplies, and improved functioning of information and logistic systems."[78] The new approach calls explicitly for a business model that encourages country ownership, invests in country-led plans, and creates sustainability through health systems improvements.

The rhetoric is right, but time will tell whether resources follow. Changing the orientation of U.S. policy and implementing a more comprehensive approach to global health challenges will be a slow and uneven process. Notably, under the proposed fiscal year 2011 budget, the FE(L)TP program would receive significant new funding. On the other hand, the Global Disease

---

77.   Department of State, "The U.S. President's Emergency Plan for AIDS Relief: Five-Year Strategy."
78.   Department of State, "Implementation of the Global Health Initiative: Consultation Document," February 2010, 4–5, www.pepfar.gov/documents/organization/136504.pdf.

Detection program annual budget is flat, and falls far short of what is needed to make significant strides toward reaching the program's full potential.[79]

Many believe that a major challenge to creating a new approach to global health in general and to expanding support for foreign capacity in infectious disease surveillance and response in particular, is a fragmented bureaucracy and the need to better harmonize U.S. global health policy. This call for greater interagency coordination in global health policy is echoed in debates about U.S. development and foreign aid policy broadly writ.[80]

It is true that there is no overarching coordinating mechanism across the major agencies; no plan for creating an integrated, interagency structure; and until the GHI, no government-wide plan for meeting global health challenges. Although the various agencies meet and discuss programs frequently, no one office or individual resolves conclusively which agency will lead on which issue. Coordination mechanisms do exist for particular disease initiatives, however. The State Department's Office of Global Aid Coordinator is the guiding agency for the many HIV/AIDS-related programs, and USAID leads in the implementation of the President's Malaria Initiative, for example. These disease-specific coordination bodies generally receive high marks for providing a strategic focus to the programs under their jurisdiction. Further, each of the major agencies involved in shaping global health policy has its own mechanism for coordination. For example, the Office of Global Health Affairs is the focal point for the global health activities of HHS and the CDC. It provides centralized administrative support for several programs described above, although it lacks budgetary authority over them.

Although improved interagency coordination is something everyone can agree on in principle, in practice there are many competing notions of how best to achieve broad coordination of U.S. global health policy and where best to locate authority to resolve issues concerning overlapping agency jurisdiction. Many call for the creation of an interagency task force to improve policy coherence chaired by a senior official in the Office of the President, the National Security Council, or the Homeland Security Council.[81] Alternatively, some favor the creation of a new cabinet-level post with responsibility over the issue of global health or health and development

79. Kaiser Family Foundation, "Budget Tracker: Status of U.S. FY 11 Funding for Key Global Health and Related Accounts," February 17, 2010, http://globalhealth.kff.org/Policy-Tracker/Administration/Actions/2010/February/01/FY11-Budget-Request.aspx.

80. See, for example, Marie Leonardo Lawson and Susan B. Epstein, "Foreign Aid Reform: Agency Coordination" (Washington, DC: Congressional Research Service, August 7, 2009), www.fas.org/sgp/crs/row/R40756.pdf.

81. See IOM, "U.S. Commitment to Global Health;" Levine, "Healthy Foreign Policy;" National Academies, "Global Health."

more broadly.[82] Under President Obama, global health matters fall under the purview of Gayle Smith, special assistant to the president and National Security Council senior director for global development, stabilization, and humanitarian assistance.

Centralization of policy might help with disputes concerning interagency power-sharing in Washington, but it is unlikely to be a panacea for improving support for, or the operational effectiveness of, overseas capacity in infectious disease control. Centralization and a common strategic framework issuing from the White House, National Security Council, or Homeland Security Council would not be without its potential costs. Centralization of global health policymaking risks pulling strategy further away from those experts who know the medical, technical, and in-country dynamics best. These experts are more likely located in Atlanta and around the world rather than inside the Washington Beltway. They have superior knowledge of programs and possibilities, an understanding of what works in different settings, and an appreciation for cost-effectiveness and sustainability. Public health professionals also stay with the issue for the long-term and have fewer short-term or political motivations for the actions they recommend. Furthermore, they have real, robust, and efficacious networks across governmental agencies, within countries, and in multilateral institutions involved in the same issue area, all of which are essential to the success of health initiatives. Furthermore, interagency coordination is probably better "in the field," that is, in-country, than it is in Washington. Most long-time infectious disease experts, be they in the DOD, CDC, or USAID are mission oriented and committed to finding ways to get the job done efficiently.[83] Both civilian and military officials point to the effective teamwork between their co-located disease detection programs in the Middle East and South America, for example.[84] Admittedly, the level of coordination varies from one country or region to the next and it may turn on personal and professional relationships, but edicts from a Washington global health czar in the name of latest health strategy is unlikely to improve this reality. Coordinated reporting mechanisms would likely help promote the most effective practices and eliminate redundancies.

---

82. See Salaam-Blyther, "Centers for Disease Control;" Maria Leonardo Lawson and Susan B. Epstein, "Foreign Aid Reform: Agency Coordination," CRS Report R40756 (Washington, DC: Congressional Research Service, August 7, 2009), www.fas.org/sgp/crs/row/R40756.pdf; F. Brian Atwood et al., "Arrested Development," *Foreign Affairs* 87, no. 6 (2008): 123–32.

83. Personal interviews, Atlanta, GA, January 29, 2010; Washington, DC, March 2, 2010.

84. Ibid.

Ironically, greater centralization and politicization of global health policy also runs the risk of reducing the political effectiveness of U.S. policy designed to improve foreign capacity in infectious disease control. One of the great political advantages global health professionals have is that they generally are not viewed as political actors. Most of those implementing U.S. infectious disease control policy are medical and public health specialists and scientists who see the first order of business as "doing good public health," and they are appreciated abroad as being extraordinarily good at what they do.[85] Indeed, in some countries, CDC is not even perceived by some of its beneficiaries as being part of the U.S. government.[86] DOD also designs its programs to correspond to the interests of the host country and with the goal of helping the host country meet its surveillance and reporting requirements under the IHR 2005.[87] Because of their reputation for doing good work well, U.S. public health officials working this issue can play a critical and early role in many conflict or postconflict situations, as they are in Iraq and Afghanistan, for example, and they can enhance relations with difficult countries that would reject a more openly political overture, as is happening in Yemen or Sudan, for instance. In short, centralization could further exclude from strategy those who know the issues the best and compromise some of the delicate but important political dividends associated with global public health initiatives.

Furthermore, harmonization in this area should not mean that U.S. policy has a single voice, only that it works in concert. U.S. infectious disease control policies are not meant to serve one policy goal, but several: national security, economic development, human rights, public diplomacy, commercial interests, and others. It is both natural and inevitable that different agencies should pursue different goals consistent with their respective core missions. For example, DOD's greatest concern is ensuring the health of its troops, protecting American borders from foreign (microbial) invasion, and promoting stability in foreign nations in which they operate. Capacity building in public health is a means to these ends. CDC, by contrast, gives pride of place to building sound medical practices and capacity abroad, thereby serving national security as a consequence. Each agency has unique strengths in health as well. CDC is considered the gold standard in epidemiological practice and countries are eager to work with it in part because it is not seen as a military or even political actor. DOD, by virtue of its logistical abilities,

---

85. Personal interview, Atlanta, GA, January 29, 2010.
86. Ibid.
87. Personal interview, Washington, DC, March 2, 2010.

can deliver health services and build capacity in regions that might be difficult or dangerous for civilians. Military-to-military cooperation is also an important pillar in its own right in good bilateral relations. Complementary mandates of the agencies involved in global public health leverage different skills and perspectives to extend the scope and performance of U.S. policies designed to improve foreign capacity in infectious disease control even at the risk of some duplication of effort and jurisdictional disputes at the margin.

Conclusion

U.S. global health policy has yet to fully match rhetoric with reality regarding strengthening overseas capacity in infectious disease surveillance and response. To do so would require a steady increase in the base funding for programs such as the GDD, FE(L)TP, and IDSR. These programs are precisely the type of long-term, system-strengthening initiatives that are the aspiration of Obama's Global Health Initiative. These programs help contain disease outbreaks; transfer technical skills in epidemiology, surveillance, and health promotion to partner countries in the developing world; and establish evidence-based technical standards and procedures that create the possibility for regional or global collaboration.[88] Many of these programs have operated quietly and effectively for years. In addition to their successes in controlling disease spread, there is substantial anecdotal evidence of the political goodwill and image promotion these programs generate. In one recent example, the People's Republic of China recognized a senior CDC epidemiologist with its highest award to a foreign national for his contribution in improving disease surveillance, data management, outbreak investigation, and international understanding.[89]

Given that the United States dedicates so much funding to particular diseases, a near-term transition to a system strengthening perspective might require a mechanism such as a set-aside of a percentage of disease-specific funding to be used for improving public health infrastructure in the developing world in core competencies that include infectious disease control and laboratory capacity. These systems will help ensure the long-run success of disease-specific initiatives. This allocation would compel programs like

---

88. Ibid., 58. See also, U.S. Congress, Senate, Committee on Appropriations, Subcommittee on Labor, Health and Human Services, Education and Related Agencies, "Prepared Testimony of Stephen Blount, director for Global Health, CDC," May 2, 2007, www.dhhs.gov/asl/testify/2007/05/t20070502a.html.
89. CDC, "Robert Fontaine Received the Friendship Award," newsletter, October 2007.

PEPFAR to move in the direction it has chosen for itself in its most recent five-year strategic plan and help move the GHI from rhetoric to reality.

Creation of an interagency committee to provide greater harmony in U.S. global health policy is potentially useful but undue centralization may be hazardous to promoting infectious disease control capacity abroad. Any new coordinating body would ideally find ways to reach out to and incorporate those technical specialists and agencies (particularly CDC and USAID) who know both the diseases and the country conditions in great detail in forming broad strategies while refraining from overtly politicizing medical experts and programs who have developed years and sometimes decades of good will as nonpolitical actors in the countries where they work. Finally, centralizing policy should avoid subordinating complex and diffuse networks of interagency and international coordination to a Washington-based political compromise that, while more uniform, may be less effective in serving the many distinctive but interrelated goals pursued through America's disease control policies.

6

CONCLUSIONS AND
FURTHER RESEARCH

This study focuses on seemingly anomalous instances of international cooperation in infectious disease control among countries with historic or present antipathies and in resource-constrained environments. It asks why these states cooperate on a matter of state security and welfare that exposes their national vulnerabilities to past or current adversaries. The answer is complex and requires drawing on several theories of international relations—realism, liberal institutionalism, and constructivism—as well as on sociological and psychological theories of intergroup and interpersonal dynamics.

Using the lens of political realism, we identify a shared compelling material interest in a transnational public good (protection from infectious diseases), appreciate how the nature of this good creates consumption externalities that further encourage cooperation, and recognize how a state might both weigh the dangers posed by pandemic disease spread against the danger of sharing sensitive information with neighboring states and rationally decide that the vulnerability presented by the former outweighs that presented by the latter. From liberal institutionalism, we recognize the importance of interdependence in drawing states into joint action for mutual gain and how the organization of cooperation must engage those actors, and ideally only those actors, with a shared vulnerability and the means and motivation to seek a solution. From constructivism and social psychology, we see the importance of identity in defining actor preferences, how antagonistic national identities might be reconfigured to form a new shared transnational identity that, though not eliminating national identity, can take precedence in certain situations and allow for cooperation in a trusted network that is scalable from interpersonal relations up to effective transnational institutions.

In explaining these important but largely unrecognized instances of interstate cooperation, each of these powerful paradigms solves a piece of the puzzle. Rather than engaging in a tired debate of which approach is rightfully the king of the hill, this book demonstrates how elements of grand theory originally created to explain international cooperation and conflict globally or universally might be blended and applied to provide a compelling explanation for unexpected, real-world cooperation occurring in different regional settings. This is particularly important today because many issues of interstate order, security, conflict, and cooperation involve actions and arrangements operating at a regional level. As Lake and Morgan note, "Regions are not simply 'little' international systems that behave in ways identical to their larger counterparts. Nor are they sui generis, understandable only through unique theories. We need general theories that incorporate regional relations."[1] This study provides one such theory of regional cooperation that applies in different settings and may have explanatory power in other regions and issue areas.

The theory of cooperation developed here suggests to both scholars and practitioners that by getting interests, institutions, and identity right (no small task), the scope of potential interstate cooperation may be greater than we presume. Given the litany of transnational problems waiting to be addressed and many transnational public goods yet to be secured, this study provides a hopeful illustration of what might be possible in issues as diverse as combating terrorism, countering weapons proliferation, sustaining natural resource commons, and preventing violations of human rights occurring across state boundaries. Each of these issues would benefit greatly by the formulation of a trusted transnational network that shared information and initiatives in common purpose.

The networked cooperation studied in this book also provided a basis for systematic comparison of the process of transnational governance. The actors involved in the three disease surveillance networks studied here include states, international organizations, national and international nongovernmental organizations, and other important private actors with considerable resources such as corporations and philanthropies. These public-private problem-solving networks are an important new development in transnational or global governance. They have generated substantial interest and opinion among scholars, but few comparative case studies leading to hypotheses

---

1.   David A. Lake and Patrick M. Morgan, "The New Regional in Security Affairs," in *Regional Orders: Building Security in a New World*, eds. David Lake and Patrick Morgan (University Park: Pennsylvania University Press, 1997), 7.

about what makes them effective in securing transnational public goods or legitimate in terms of their democratic accountability.

The second contribution of this book is both an account of how these public-private entities operate and a distillation from the cases of the factors that appear to make them both effective in providing transnational public goods and legitimate to domestic and international constituencies. The goal here is to generate hypotheses for further scholarly investigation, testing, and refinement and to provide a plausible framework for thinking about the structure and function of a successful transnational public-private network for practitioners. This single study is not conclusive on either score, of course, but it perhaps provides a well-reasoned platform for further scholarship and a checklist of factors practitioners might consider in designing and operating transnational networks in their areas of expertise.

This dimension of the study suggests that interstate cooperation is a necessary condition for creating an effective transnational network in that state actors are the indispensable and authoritative conduit between international negotiations and national implementation. Interstate cooperation, in turn, depends on the correct alignment of interests, institutions, and ideas. In addition, the cases suggest at least five other key variables: actions congruent with international norms and the practice of international organizations; policies that strengthen the capacity of each member and the partnership as a whole; partnership roles that correspond to the particular strengths and capacities of the types of actors involved; formal plans and concrete goals and responsibilities, but not arbitrary or politically inspired timetables so as to allow for some flexibility and adaptability in programs and procedures; and a committed core and multiple auxiliary sources of financial supporters. The cases also suggest key variables contributing to the legitimacy of transnational public-private problem-solving networks defined in terms of democratic accountability. The five factors positively correlated with network legitimacy include inclusive membership to allow for voice by many parties with a stake in the outcome of decisions, the equitable exercise of power as reflected in the key institutions and internal rules of the transnational organization, accountability of all parties to one or preferably several empowering authorities and to affected populations, organizational transparency ideally from multiple sources of reporting, and deliberative and consensual decision making.

The third major area of inquiry in this book is the impact and potential of national policies as a potential complement to regional and global efforts to control infectious disease. Specifically, U.S. public health diplomacy in the support of foreign capacity for infectious disease surveillance and response is examined. The United States, as a global leader in the relevant technologies and with a legacy of success in disease eradication and control, has an important but indirect role to play in promoting regional cooperation in this area. Strengthening foreign capacity in infectious disease control is vital to U.S. security and economic interests and an area of unsurpassed potential for improving its foreign relations on a bilateral, regional, and global basis. Simply put, capacity building abroad in infectious disease surveillance and response is an area ripe for the pursuit of America's enlightened self-interest.

U.S. policies in this area are significant, if little known, and this book outlines some of the key players, policy initiatives, and their impacts. Given the seriousness of the threat posed by the spread of infectious disease and the vast potential for goodwill to be had from U.S. support for overseas surveillance and response capacity, however, this policy area requires greater U.S. commitment of funds and expertise, especially in view of America's growing global public health expenditures generally. At their current levels, U.S. support for foreign capacity in infectious disease control is shortchanging American interests. This study recommends a significant increase in the size of U.S. programs devoted to this challenge. In the context of overall U.S. global health expenditures, even an increased expenditure on foreign capacity for infectious disease control would be only a small fraction of America's international public health budget but would deliver significant security and diplomatic returns on the investment.

With an expansion of policy will come a greater need for interagency coordination. In harmonizing U.S. policies in support of foreign capacity in infectious disease control, policy elites should recognize the distinctive security, commercial, developmental, diplomatic, and humanitarian goals served by agencies currently involved in this policy arena, however. Further, policy reform should avoid disenfranchising field experts from the formulation of a Washington-led consensus.

Future Research

A useful study should unearth more questions than it resolves. It is hoped that readers have their own ideas of how the ideas offered here might be best used to explore issues in international cooperation, transnational governance, and American global health diplomacy, but let me suggest a few potential paths of further investigation.

One open question is the extent to which cooperation in this aspect of public health can spillover into related functional issues or lead to new forms of transnational political cooperation. The hope that health is the leading edge of peace is neither confirmed nor negated in this study, but the organizations studied are all relatively new entities. Thus far, the transnational networks studied here have generated some related cooperation in other health matters and in natural disaster response and have led to the initiation of a new NGO of global scope that is just beginning to link these networks together in common purpose. More time and further investigation would tell us more about whether these networks or newly emerging others, such as the South Africa Center for Infectious Disease Surveillance, could secure a wider cooperation that promotes regional stability.

For those most interested in cooperation through health, this study may be a useful addition to the literature, but it is neither the first nor (one hopes) the last word on the role of health in interstate cooperation. This study looks at a particular form of institutionalized transborder regional cooperation. But health can be used in other ways to encourage or facilitate international cooperation and conflict resolution. Health has the power to convene actors in a common purpose, to signal the possibility of rapprochement between long-standing adversaries, and as a positive dimension of larger interstate dynamic. Recent exchanges between North and South Korea on maternal and child care,[2] between North Korea and American nongovernmental organizations on drug-resistant tuberculosis diagnosis,[3] between Turkey and Armenia on avian influenza,[4] and between the EU and Libya on infectious disease control,[5] are but a few of the intriguing examples of the role of health initiatives as an icebreaker in traditionally hostile relations. Bilateral health cooperation is also an important pillar of great power relations[6] and an emerging dimension of South-South cooperation.[7] These forms of health diplomacy are not the focus of this study, but are equally important topics for students of international cooperation.

---

2.   Stephanie Nebehay, "Health Project Helps North-South Korean Ties: WHO," *Reuters*, March 4, 2010, www.reuters.com/assests/print?aid=USTRE62336I20100304.

3.   Global Health and Security Initiative, "New Tuberculosis Lab Developed in North Korea with Support from NTI's Global Health and Security Initiative," press release, February 25, 2010 (Washington, DC: Nuclear Threat Initiative, 2010), www.nti.org/c_press/c2_pressreleases.html.

4.   Personal interview, Atlanta, GA, July 10, 2009.

5.   "EU-Libya Cooperation Deal on Infectious Diseases," *ANSAmed*, November 20, 2009.

6.   See, for example, "China, USG Deepen Medical, Science, Technology Cooperation," *SinoCast China Business Daily News*, December 5, 2008; The White House, "U.S.-Russian Cooperation in Public Health and Medical Sciences," (Washington, DC: Executive Office of the President, July 6, 2009).

7.   See, for example, "India, Brazil to Cooperate in Health R&D, IPR, Traditional Medicine," *United News of India*, July 28, 2008.

One of the bolder assertions here is that the explanation for the dynamics of regional, transnational cooperation in these settings and in this issue area may apply in other settings and to other transnational problems. The basis for this belief rests on the fact that the cases described here are, to a degree, least likely cases of interstate cooperation. They are unlikely instances of cooperation, first, because the most successful cases involve parties in conflict or without a history of cooperative interactions, and, second, because the issue area (infectious disease control) is particularly vexatious in that it requires a state to share information revealing the vulnerabilities of its population and the weaknesses of its institutions to another state that is not a trusted partner. As a result, I suggest that if traditional adversaries can cooperate in an area that presents a potential threat to a government or to the state itself, perhaps other transnational issues and other groups of actors are amenable to finding cooperative solutions by aligning their interests, institutions, and identities. This is not to suggest that the process is easy; it is not. But it may be possible. Analyses of other attempts at transnational cooperation, both successful and unsuccessful, will tell if this assertion is well founded.

For those interested in questions of transnational or networked governance and problem solving, this study offers specific empirically based hypotheses on what makes this new form of governance effective and legitimate. If plausible, the hypotheses should be tested and refined. Do the suggested necessary and facilitating variables contributing to effective and legitimate governance in these cases evince themselves in other instances of successful transnational governance that seek to deliver public goods and are they absent in unsuccessful cases? Are other factors important to consider in different contexts and why? Furthermore, might a larger statistical study help us understand the interaction and relative importance among the variables cited in this study?

Finally, with regard to national, specifically U.S. foreign policies in support of foreign capacity in infectious disease surveillance and response, it bears watching to see if the President's new Global Health Initiative translates into greater, more comprehensive, and better coordinated support for strengthening infectious disease control systems abroad as a first line of defense for America's security and welfare and as a meaningful demonstration of America's commitment to improving the health and well-being of people everywhere.

BIBLIOGRAPHY

Contributing to One World, One Health: A Strategic Framework for Reducing the Risks of Infectious Diseases at the Animal-Human-Ecosystems Interface. Consultation document. Rome: Food and Agriculture Organization, World Organization for Animal Health (OIE), World Health Organization, United Nations Influenza Coordination, United Nations Children's Fund (UNICEF), and the World Bank, 2008. www.fao.org/docrep/011/aj137e/aj137e00.htm.

Adams, Vincanne, and Thomas Novotny. "Global Health Diplomacy." Working paper, Global Health Sciences, University of California, San Francisco, January 16, 2007.

Aginam, Obijiofor. *Global Health Governance: International Law and Public Health in a Divided World.* Toronto: University of Toronto Press, 2005.

Armed Forces Health Surveillance Center. "Global Emerging Infections Surveillance and Response Systems." Washington, DC: U.S. Department of Defense. www.afhsc.mil/geisPartners.

Arrow, Kenneth. *The Limits of Organization.* New York: W. W. Norton, 1974.

Atwood, F. Brian, M. Peter McPherson, and Andrew Natsios. "Arrested Development." *Foreign Affairs* 87, no. 6 (2008): 123–32.

Barrett, Scott. *Why Cooperate? The Incentive to Supply Global Public Goods.* New York: Oxford University Press, 2007.

Berlinguer, Giovanni. "Health and Equity as a Primary Global Goal." *Development* 42, no. 2 (1999): 12–16.

Bloom, William. *Personal Identity, National Identity, and International Relations.* Cambridge: Cambridge University Press, 1990.

Bond, Katherine. "Promoting Trans-National Collaboration in Disease Surveillance and Control." Presentation, Rockefeller Foundation Africa Regional Office, Nairobi, Kenya, April 28, 2009. www.rockfound.org/about_us/speeches/042809swine_flu_k_bond.shtml.

Bonventre, Eugene V., Kathleen H. Hicks, and Stacy M. Okutani. "U.S. National Security and Global Health: An Analysis of Global Health Engagement by the U.S. Department of Defense." Washington, DC: Center for Strategic and International Studies, April 2009. http://csis.org/files/publication/090421_Bonventre_USNationalSecurity_Rev.pdf.

Borzel, Tania A., and Thomas Risse. "Public-Private Partnerships: Effective and Legitimate Tools of Transnational Governance." In *Complex Sovereignty: Reconstituting Political Authority in the Twenty-First Century,* edited by Edgar Grande and Louis W. Pauly, 195–216. Toronto: University of Toronto Press, 2005.

Bradach, Jeffrey L., and Robert G. Eccles. "Price, Authority, and Trust: From Ideal Types to Plural Forms." *Annual Review of Sociology* 15, no. 1 (1989): 97–118.

Brewer, Marilynn B. "When Contact Is Not Enough: Social Identity and Intergroup Cooperation." *International Journal of Intercultural Relations* 20, no. 3/4 (1996): 291–303.

Brower, Jennifer, and Peter Chalk. *The Global Threat of New and Reemerging Infectious Diseases: Reconciling U.S. National Security and Public Health Policies.* Santa Monica, CA: RAND Corporation, 2003.

Buse, Kent, and Andrew Harmer. "Power to the Partners? The Politics of Public-Private Health Partnerships." *Development* 47, no. 2 (2004): 49–56.

Buse, Kent, and Gill Walt. "Global Public-Private Partnerships: Part I, A New Development in Health." *Bulletin of the World Health Organization* 78, no. 4 (2000): 1–19.

———. "The World Health Organization and Global Public-Private Health Partnerships: In Search of Good Global Governance." In *Public-Private Partnerships: Theory and Practice in International Perspective*, edited by Stephen P. Osborne, 169–96. London: Routledge, 2000.

———. "Globalisation and Multilateral Public-Private Health Partnerships: Issues for Health Policy." In *Health Policy in a Globalising World*, edited by Kelley Lee, Susan Fustukian, and Kent Buse, 41–62. Cambridge: Cambridge University Press, 2002.

―――. "Global Public-Private Partnerships: Part II, What Are the Health Issues for Global Governance." *Bulletin of the World Health Organization* 78, no. 5 (2005): 699–709. www.who.int/bulletin/archives/78(5)699.pdf.

Buse, Kent, Nick Drager, Suzanne Fustukian, and Kelley Lee. "Globalisation and Health Policy: Trends and Opportunities." In *Health Policy in a Globalising World*, edited by Kelley Lee, Susan Fustukian, and Kent Buse, 251–280. Cambridge: Cambridge University Press, 2002.

Calain, Phillipe. "Exploring the International Arena of Global Public Health Surveillance." *Health Policy and Planning* 22, no. 1 (2007): 2–12.

―――. "From the Field Side of the Binoculars: A Different View on Global Public Health Surveillance." *Health Policy Planning* 22, no. 1 (2007): 13–20.

Chayes, Abram, Antonia Handler Chayes, and Ronald B. Mitchell. "Managing Compliance: A Comparative Perspective." In *Engaging Countries: Strengthening Compliance with International Environmental Accords*, edited by Edith Brown Weiss and Harold K. Jacobsen, 39–62. Cambridge, MA: MIT Press, 1998.

Chen, Lincoln, Tim Evans, and Richard Cash. "Health as a Global Public Good." In *Global Public Goods: International Cooperation in the 21st Century*, edited by Inge Kaul, Isabelle Grunberg, and Mark A. Sterns, 284–305. New York: Oxford University Press, 1999.

Clinton, Hillary Rodham. "Remarks on Human Rights Agenda for the 21st Century." Georgetown University, Washington, DC, December 14, 2009.

Commission on Macroeconomics and Health. *Investing in Health*. Geneva: World Health Organization, 2003.

Cronin, Bruce. *Community under Anarchy: Transnational Identity and the Evolution of Cooperation*. New York: Columbia University Press, 1999.

Decker, K. C., and Keith Holtermann. "The Role for Exercises in Senior Policy Pandemic Influenza Preparedness." *Journal of Homeland Security and Emergency Management* 6, no. 1 (2009): 1–15. doi:10.2202/1547-7355.1521.

Deeg, Richard, and Mary O'Sullivan. "The Political Economy of Global Financial Capital." *World Politics* 61, no. 4 (October 2009): 731–63.

Denny, Colleen D., and Ezekial J. Emanuel. "U.S. Health Aid beyond PEPFAR: The Mother and Child Campaign." *Journal of the American Medical Association* 300, no. 17 (November 2008): 2048–51.

Djelic, Marie-Laurie, and Kerstin Sahlin-Andersen. "Introduction: A World of Governance: The Rise of Transnational Regulation." In *Transnational*

Governance: Institutional Dynamics of Regulation, edited by Marie-Laurie Djelic and Kerstin Sahlin-Andersen, 1–28. Cambridge: Cambridge University Press, 2006.

Dodgson, Richard, Kelley Lee, and Nick Drager. "Global Health Governance: A Conceptual Review." In *Global Health Governance: Key Issues*, edited by Kelley Lee. Westport, CT: Greenwood Press, 2000.

———. *Global Health Governance: A Conceptual Review*. Geneva: World Health Organization and London School of Hygiene and Tropical Medicine, 2002.

Fearon, James D. "Domestic Political Audiences and the Escalation of International Disputes." *American Political Science Review* 88, no. 3 (1994): 577–92.

Feldbaum, Harley. "U.S. Global Health and Security Policy." Washington, DC: Center for Strategic and International Studies Global Health Policy Center, April 2009. http://csis.org/files/media/csis/pubs/090420_feldbaum_usglobalhealth.pdf.

Feldbaum, Harley, Preeti Patel, Egbert Sondrop, and Kelley Lee. "Global Health and National Security: The Need for Critical Engagement." Unpublished manuscript, Center on Global Change and Health, London School of Hygiene and Tropical Medicine, 2004.

Fidler, David P. "Architecture amidst Anarchy: Global Health's Quest for Governance." *Global Health Governance* 1, no. 1 (January 2007): 1–17.

———. "Reflections on the Revolution in Health and Foreign Policy." *Bulletin of the World Health Organization* 85, no. 3 (2007): 243–44.

Fisher, Julie E., Eric Lief, Vidal Seegobin, and Jen Kates. "U.S. Global Health Policies: Mapping the United States Engagement in Global Public Health." Menlo Park, CA: Kaiser Family Foundation, August 2009. www.kff.org/globalhealth/upload/7958.pdf.

Fisher, Ronald J. *The Social Psychology of Intergroup and International Conflict Resolution*. New York: Springer-Verlag, 1990.

Food and Agriculture Organization. *Global Programme for the Prevention and Control of Highly Pathogenic Avian Influenza Report*. Rome: Food and Agriculture Organization, 2008.

Garrett, Laurie, and Kammerle Schneider. "Global Health: Getting It Right." In *Health and Development*, edited by Anna Gati and Andrea Boggio. New York: Palgrave Macmillan, 2009.

Garrett, Laurie. *The Coming Plague: Newly Emerging Diseases in a World out of Balance*. New York: Penguin, 1995.

Gavlak, Dale. "Catching Outbreaks Wherever They Occur." *World Health Organization Bulletin* 87, no. 10 (October 2009): 733–804. who.int/bulletin/volumes/87/10/09-031009/en/. doi:10.2471/BLT.03.001009.

George, Alexander L. *Bridging the Gap: Theory and Practice in Foreign Policy*. Washington, DC: U.S. Institute of Peace Press, 2003.

George, Alexander L., and Andrew Bennett. *Case Studies and Theory Development in the Social Sciences*. Cambridge, MA: Massachusetts Institute of Technology Press, 2005.

Global Health and Security Initiative. "New Tuberculosis Lab Developed in North Korea with Support from NTI's Global Health and Security Initiative." Press release. February 25, 2010. Washington, DC: Nuclear Threat Initiative, 2010. www.nti.org/c_press/release_North%20Korea_022510.pdf.

Gomez, Eduardo. "Stop Fighting Viruses, Start Treating People." *Foreign Policy*, January 27, 2010. www.foreignpolicy.com/articles/2010/01/27/stop_fighting_viruses_start_treating_people.

Grande, Edgar, and Louis W. Pauly. "Complex Sovereignty and the Emergence of Transnational Authority." In *Complex Sovereignty: Reconstituting Political Authority in the Twenty-First Century*, edited by Edgar Grande and Louis W. Pauly. Toronto: University of Toronto Press, 2005.

———. "Reconstituting Political Authority: Sovereignty, Effectiveness, and Legitimacy in a Transnational Order." In *Complex Sovereignty: Reconstituting Political Authority in the Twenty-First Century*, edited by Edgar Grande and Louis W. Pauly, 3–21. Toronto: University of Toronto Press, 2005.

Gresham, Louise, Assad Ramlawi, Julie Briski, Mariah Richardson, and Terence Taylor. "Trust Across Borders: Responding to the H1N1 Influenza in the Middle East." *Biosecurity and Bioterrorism: Biodefense Strategy, Practice, and Science* 7, no. 4 (2009): 399–404. doi:10.1089/bsp.2009.0034.

Hafner-Burton, Emilie M., Miles Kahler, and Alexander H. Montgomery. "Networked Analysis for International Relations." *International Organization* 63 (Summer 2009): 559–92.

Hannerz, Ulf. *Transnational Connections: Culture, People, Places*. London: Routledge, 1996.

Hass, Ernst. *The Uniting of Europe: Political, Social, and Economic Sources 1950–1957*. Stanford, CA: Stanford University Press, 1958.

Hass, Peter M. "Knowledge, Power and International Policy Coordination." *International Organization* 46, no. 1 (1992): 1–35.

Heymann, David, and Guenael Rodier. "Global Surveillance, National Surveillance, and SARS." *Emerging Infectious Diseases* 10, no. 2 (2004). www.medscape.com/viewarticle/467371.

Hurd, Ian. "Legitimacy and Authority in International Politics." *International Organization* 53, no. 2 (1999): 379–408.

Huxham, Chris, and Siv Vangen. "What Makes Partnerships Work?" In *Public-Private Partnerships: Theory and Practice in International Perspective*, edited by Stephen P. Osborne, 293–310. London: Routledge, 2000.

Ikerd, John E. "Rethinking the Economics of Self-Interest." Conference paper presented at the Organization for Comparative Markets, Omaha, NE, September 1999.

Institute of Medicine (IOM). *Review of the DoD-GEIS Influenza Programs.* Washington, DC: National Academies Press, 2008.

———. "The U.S. Commitment to Global Health: Recommendations for the New Administration." Washington, DC: National Academies Press, 2009.

Kaiser Family Foundation. "U.S. Global Health Policy, The U.S. Government's Global Health Policy Architecture: Structure Programs, and Funding." Menlo Park, CA: Kaiser Family Foundation, April 2009. www.kff.org/globalhealth/upload/7881.pdf.

Kapp, Lawrence, and Don J. Jansen. "The Role of the Department of Defense During a Flu Pandemic." CRS Report R40619. Washington, DC: Congressional Research Service, June 2009. www.fas.org/sgp/crs/natsec/R40619.pdf.

Kates, Jen. "The U.S. Global Health Initiative: Overview and Budget Analysis." Menlo Park, CA: Kaiser Family Foundation, December 2009. http://kff.org/globalhealth/upload/8009.pdf.

Katzenstein, Peter, ed. *The Culture of National Security.* Princeton, NJ: Princeton University Press, 1996.

Keck, Margaret, and Kathryn Sikkink. *Activists beyond Borders: Advocacy Networks in International Politics.* Ithaca, NY: Cornell University Press, 1998.

Keohane, Robert. "Accountability in World Politics." *Scandinavian Political Studies* 29, no. 2 (2006): 75–87.

Keohane, Robert, and Joseph Nye Jr. "Transnational Relations and World Politics: An Introduction." In *Transnational Relations and World Politics*, edited by Robert Keohane and Joseph Nye Jr., xi–xvi. Cambridge, MA: Harvard University Press, 1971.

———. *Power and Interdependence*, 3rd ed. New York: Longman, 2000.

Kickbusch, Ilona, and Jonathan Quick. "Partnership for Health in the 21st Century." *World Health Statistics Quarterly* 51 (1998): 68–74.

Kickbusch, Ilona, Gaudenz Silberschmidt, and Paulo Buss. "Global Health Diplomacy: The Need for New Perspectives, Strategic Approaches and Skills in Global Health." *World Health Organization Bulletin* 85, no. 3 (March 1987): 161–244. www.who.int/bulletin/volumes/85/3/06-039222/en/.

Kimball, Ann Marie, Melinda Moore, Howard Matthew French, Yuzo Arima, Kumnuan Ungchusak, Suwit Wibulpolprasert, Terence Taylor, Sok Touch, and Alex Leventhal. "Regional Infectious Disease Surveillance Networks and their Potential to Facilitate the Implementation of International Health Regulations." *Medical Clinics North America* 92 (2008): 1459–71. doi:10.1016/j.mcna.2008.06.001.

King, Gary, and Langche Zang. "Improving Forecasts of State Failure." *World Politics* 53, no. 4 (July 2001): 623–58. doi:10.1353/wp.2001.0018.

King, Gary, Robert Keohane, and Sidney Verba. *Designing Social Inquiry*. Princeton, NJ: Princeton University Press, 1994.

Klijn, Erik-Hans, and Geert R. Teisman. "Governing Public-Private Partnerships." In *Public-Private Partnerships: Theory and Practice in International Perspective*, edited by Stephen P. Osborne, 84–102. London: Routledge, 2000.

Kydd, Andrew H. *Trust and Mistrust in International Relations.* Princeton, NJ: Princeton University Press, 2005.

Lake, David A., and Patrick M. Morgan. "The New Regional in Security Affairs." In *Regional Orders: Building Security in a New World*, edited by David Lake and Patrick Morgan, 3–19. University Park: Pennsylvania University Press, 1997.

Lane, Christel. "Introduction: Theories and Issues in the Study of Trust." In *Trust Within and Between Organizations*, edited by Christel Lane and Reinhard Bachmann, 1–30. Oxford: Oxford University Press, 1998.

Lassman, Peter, and Ronald Speirs, eds. *Weber: Political Writings.* Cambridge: Cambridge University Press, 1994.

Lawson, Marie Leonardo, and Susan B. Epstein. "Foreign Aid Reform: Agency Coordination." CRS Report R40756. Washington, DC: Congressional Research Service, August 7, 2009. www.fas.org/sgp/crs/row/R40756.pdf.

Lee, Kelley. "Globalization: A New Agenda for Health." In *International Cooperation in Health*, edited by Martin McKee, Paul Garner, and Robin Stott, 13–30. Oxford: Oxford University Press, 2001.

———. *Globalization and Health*. New York: Palgrave Macmillan, 2003.

Lee, Kelley, and Derek Yach. "Globalization and Health." In *International Public Health: Disease, Programs, Systems and Policies*, edited by Michael H. Merson, Robert E. Black, and Anne J. Mills, 681–708. Sudbury, MA: Jones and Bartlett Publishers, 2006.

Lee, Kelley, Susan Fustukian, and Kent Buse. "An Introduction to Global Health Policy." In *Health Policy in a Globalising World*, edited by Kelley Lee, Susan Fustukian, and Kent Buse, 3–17. Cambridge: Cambridge University Press, 2002.

Levanthal, Alex, and Dany Cohen. "Surveillance Systems in Practice." Presentation, International Meeting on Emerging Disease and Response 2009, Vienna, Austria, February 15, 2009. www.imed.isid.org/IMED2009/preliminary_schedule.shtml.

Levine, Ruth. "Healthy Foreign Policy: Bringing Coherence to the Global Health Agenda." In *The White House and the World: A Global Development Agenda for the Next U.S. President*, edited by Nancy Birdsall. Washington, DC: Center for Global Development, 2008.

Lewis, J. David, and Andrew Weigert. "Trust as a Social Concept." *Social Forces* 63, no. 4 (June 1985): 967–85.

Lister, Sarah A., and C. Stephen Redhead. "The 2009 Influenza Pandemic: An Overview." CRS Report R40554. Washington, DC: Congressional Research Service, September 10, 2009. http://assets.opencrs.com/rpts/R40554_20090910.pdf.

Lukwago, Luswa, Miriam Nanyunja, Joseph Wamala, Mugaga Malimbo, William Mbabazi, Anne Gasasira, Monica Musenero, Wondimagegnehu Alemu, Helen Perry, Peter Nsubuga, and Ambrose Talisuna. "The Implementation of Integrated Disease Surveillance and Response in Uganda: A Review of Progress and Challenges between 2001 and 2007." Unpublished internal report. Kampala: Ministry of Health of Uganda and WHO Uganda Country Office.

MacLean, Sandra J. "Microbes, Mad Cows, and Militaries: Exploring the Links between Health and Security." *Security Dialogue* 39, no. 5 (2008): 475–94.

MacQueen, Graeme, and Joanna Santa-Barbara. "Peacebuilding through Health Initiatives." *British Medical Journal* 321 (2000): 293–96.

Mathers, Colin D., and Dejan Loncar. "Projections of Global Mortality and Burden of Disease for 2002 to 2030." *PLOS Medicine* 3, no. 11 (2006): 2111–30.

Mayntz, Renate. "From Government to Governance: Political Steering in Modern Societies." Paper presented at the Summer Academy of International Public Policy, Wuerzburg, September 7–11, 2003.

Mboera, L. E. G. et al. "Technical Report: East African Integrated Surveillance Network, 2001-2004." Dar es Salaam, Tanzania: National Institute for Medical Research, November 2004.

McInnes, Colin J. "Looking Beyond the National Interest: Restructuring the Debate on Health and Foreign Policy." *Medical Journal of Australia* 180 (February 16, 2004): 168–70.

McKee, Martin, Paul Gardner, and Robin Scott. "Introduction." In *International Co-operation in Health*. Oxford: Oxford University Press, 2001.

———, ed. *International Co-operation and Health.* Oxford: Oxford University Press, 2001.

McQuaid, Ronald W. "The Theory of Partnerships. Why Have Partnerships?" in *Public-Private Partnerships: Theory and Practice in International Perspective*, edited by Stephen P. Osborne, 9–35. London: Routledge, 2000.

Mekong Basin Disease Surveillance Cooperation (MBDSC). "Memorandum of Understanding Among the Health Ministries of the Six Mekong Countries on the Mekong Basin Disease Surveillance (MBDS) Project." Memorandum. Nonthaburi, Thailand: MBDSC, 2001.

———. "The Extension of Memorandum of Understanding among the Health Ministries of the Six Mekong Countries on the Mekong Basin Disease Surveillance (MBDS) Project." Memorandum. Nonthaburi, Thailand: MBDSC, 2007.

———. *Action Plan (2008–2013).* Nonthaburi, Thailand: MBDSC, 2008.

Meltzer, Martin I., Nancy J. Cox, and Keiji Fukuda. "The Economic Impact of Pandemic Influenza in the United States: Priorities for Intervention." *Emerging Infectious Diseases* 5, no. 5 (1999): 659–71, www.cdc.gov/ncidod/eid/vol5no5/meltzer.htm.

Mercer, Jonathan. "Anarchy and Identity." *International Organization* 49, no. 2 (Spring 1995): 229–52.

M'ikanatha., Nkuchia M., Ruth Lynfield, Chris A. Van Beneden, and Henriette de Valk, ed. *Infectious Disease and Surveillance.* Malden, MA: Blackwell Publishing, 2007.

Mitrany, David. *A Working Peace System. An Argument for the Functional Development of International Organization.* Chicago: University of Chicago Press, 1943.

Moodie, Michael, and William J. Taylor Jr. "Contagion and Conflict: Health as a Global Security Challenge." Report of the Chemical and Biological Arms Control Institute and the Center for Strategic and International Studies, International Security Programs." Washington, DC: Center for Strategic and International Studies, 2000.

Morgenthau, Hans J. *Politics among Nations: The Struggle for Power and Peace*, 3rd ed. New York: Alfred A. Knopf, 1960.

Murphy, Craig. "Global Governance: Poorly Done and Poorly Understood." In *The Global Governance Reader*, edited by Rorden Wilkinson, 90–104. New York: Routledge, 2005.

National Intelligence Council. "The Global Infectious Disease Threat and Its Implications for the United States." NIE 99-17D. Washington, DC: National Intelligence Council, 2000. http://dni.gov/nic/special_globalinfectious.html.

Newton, Kenneth. "Social and Political Trust." In *The Oxford Handbook of Political Behavior*, edited by Russell J. Dalton and Hans-Dieter Klingemann, 342–61. Oxford: Oxford University Press, 2007.

Nishtar, Sania. "Public-Private 'Partnerships' in Health: A Global Call to Action." *Health Policy Research and Systems* 2, no. 5 (2004): 5–11. www.health-policy-systems.com/content/2/1/5.

Nye, Joseph. Smart Power: *The Means to Succeed in World Politics.* New York: Public Affairs, 2005.

Palese, Peter. "Science." Panel session at CFR Symposium on Pandemic Influenza: Science, Economics, and Foreign Policy, Council on Foreign Relations, New York, October 16, 2009. www.cfr.org/project/1442/cfr_symposium_on_pandemic_influenza.html.

Parsons, Talcott. *The Social System.* London: Routledge and Kegan Paul, 1951.

Payne, Sarah. "Globalization, Governance, and Health." In *Governance, Globalization and Public Policy*, edited by Patricia Kennett, 151–172. Cheltenham, UK: Edward Elgar, 2008.

Perry, Helen N., Sharon M. McDonnell, Wondimagegnehu Alemu, Peter Nsubuga, Stella Chungong, Mac W. Otten Jr., Paul S. Lusamba-dikassa, and Stephen B. Thacker. "Planning an Integrated Disease Surveillance and Response System: A Matrix of Skills and Activities," *BMC Medicine* 5, no. 24 (August 15, 2007): 24–32.

Peterson, Susan. "Epidemic Disease and National Security." *Security Studies* 12, no. 2 (2002): 43–81.

Price-Smith, Andrew T. *The Health of Nations: Infectious Disease, Environmental Change, and Their Effects on National Security*. Cambridge, MA: MIT Press, 2002.

———. *Contagion and Chaos: Disease Ecology and National Security in the Era of Globalization*. Cambridge, MA: MIT Press, 2009.

Putnam, Robert. *Making Democracy Work: Civic Tradition in Modern Italy*. Princeton, NJ: Princeton University Press, 1994.

Ravishankar, Nirmala, Paul Gubbins, Rebecca J. Cooley, Katherine Leach-Kemon, Catherine M. Michaud, Dean T. Jamison, and Christopher J. L. Murray. "Financing Global Health: Tracking Development Assistance for Health from 1990 to 2007." *The Lancet* 373, no. 9681 (June 20, 2009): 2113–24.

Reich, Michael R. "Introduction: Public-Private Partnerships for Public Health." In *Public-Private Partnerships for Public Health*, edited by Michael R. Reich, 1–18. Harvard Series on Population and International Health. Cambridge, MA: Harvard Center for Population and Development Studies, 2002.

———, ed. *Public-Private Partnerships for Public Health*. Harvard Series on Population and International Health. Cambridge, MA: Harvard Center for Population and Development Studies, 2002.

Reinicke, Wolfgang H., and Francis Deng. *Critical Choices. United Nations, Networks and the Future of Global Governance*. Ottawa: IDRC Publishers, 2000.

Rhodes, Rod A. W. *Understanding Governance: Policy Networks, Governance, Reflexivity, and Accountability*. Basingstoke: Macmillan, 1997.

Richter, Judith. "Public-Private Partnerships for Health: A Trend with No Alternatives." *Development* 47, no. 2 (2004): 43–48.

Rischard, Jean-François. "Global Issue Networks: Desperate Times Deserve Innovative Measures." *The Washington Quarterly* 26, no. 1 (2003): 17–33.

Risse, Thomas. "Transnational Governance and Legitimacy." Unpublished paper, Center for Transatlantic Foreign and Security Policy, Otto Suhr Institute of Political Science, Frie Universitat Berlin, February 2, 2004.

Rosenau, Pauline Vaillancourt. "The Strengths and Weaknesses of Public-Private Policy Partnerships." In *Public-Private Policy Partnerships*, edited by Pauline Vaillancourt Rosenau, 217–242. Cambridge, MA: MIT Press, 2000.

Ruggie, John Gerard. "Reconstituting the Global Public Domain: Issues, Actors, and Practices." Faculty Research Working Paper Series, JFK School of Government. Cambridge, MA: Harvard University, July 2004.

Sako, Mari. *Prices, Quality and Trust: Inter-Firm Relations in Britain and Japan.* Cambridge: Cambridge University Press, 1992.

Salaam-Blyther, Tiaji. "Centers for Disease Control and Prevention Global Health Programs: FY2001–FY2010." CRS Report 128822. Washington, DC: Congressional Research Service, August 2009. http://fpc.state.gov/documents/organization/128822.pdf.

Schäferhoff, Marco, Sabine Campe, and Christopher Kaan. "Transnational Public-Private Partnerships in International Relations: Making Sense of Concepts, Research Frameworks, and Results." *International Studies Review* 11, no. 3 (2009): 451–74. doi:10.1111/j.1468-2486.2009.00869.x.

Scharpf, Fritz W. "Introduction: The Problem-Solving Capacity of Multi-Level Governance." *Journal of European Public Policy* 4, no. 4 (1997): 520–38.

Schneider, Carmen Hackel. "Global Public Health and International Relations: Pressing Issues—Evolving Governance." *Australian Journal of International Affairs* 62, no. 1 (March 2008): 94–106.

Sikkink, Katherine, and Jackie Smith. "Infrastructure for Change: Transnational Organizations, 1953–93." In *Restructuring World Politics: Transnational Social Movements, Networks, and Norms*, edited by Sanjeev Khagram, James V. Riker, and Kathryn Sikkink, 24–46. Minneapolis: University of Minnesota Press, 2002.

Simmel, Georg. *The Philosophy of Money*. London: Routledge & Kegan Paul, 1978.

Skinner, Harvey, Ziad Abdeen, Hani Abdeen, Phil Aber, Mohammad Al-Masril, Joseph Attias, Karen B Avraham, Rivka Carmi, Catherine Chalin, Ziad El Nasser, Manaf Hijazi, Rema Othman Jebara, Moien Kanaan, Hillel Pratt, Firas Raad, Yehudah Roth, A Paul Williams, and Arnold Noyek. "Promoting Arab and Israeli Cooperation: Peacebuilding through Health Initiatives." *The Lancet* 365 (April 2, 2005): 1247–77.

Smith, Richard, David Woodward, Arnab Acharya, Robert Beaglehole, and Nick Drager. "Communicable Disease Control: A Global Public Good Perspective." *Health Policy and Planning* 15, no. 5 (2004): 271–78.

Tajfel, Henri. "Experiments in Intergroup Discrimination." *Scientific American* 223 (1970): 96–102.

Tajfel, Henri, and John C. Turner. "The Social Identity Theory of Intergroup Behavior." In *Psychology of Intergroup Relations*, edited by Stephen Worchel and William Austin, 7–24. Chicago: Nelson Hall, 1986.

The White House. "Statement by the President on Global Health Initiative." Washington, DC: Executive Office of the President, May 5, 2009. www.whitehouse.gov/the-press-office/statement-president-global-health-initiative.

———. "Memorandum of Understanding on Cooperation in the Field of Public Health and Medical Sciences." Fact Sheet. Washington, DC: Executive Office of the President, July 6, 2009. www.whitehouse.gov/the-press-office/fact-sheet-memorandum-understanding-cooperation-field-public-health-and-medical-sci.

———. "National Strategy for Countering Biological Threats." Presidential Directive. Letter of transmittal. Washington, DC: Executive Office of the President, November 2009. www.whitehouse.gov/sites/default/files/National_Strategy_for_Countering_BioThreats.pdf.

———. *National Security Strategy of the United States of America, May 2010.* Washington, DC: Executive Office of the President, 2010. www.whitehouse.gov/sites/default/files/rss_viewr/national_security_strategy.pdf.

———. Office of Science and Technology Policy. "Addressing the Threat of Emerging Infectious Diseases." Washington, DC: Executive Office of the President, June 12, 1996, www.fas.org/irp/offdocs/pdd_ntsc7.htm.

———. Office of the Vice President. "Vice President Announces Policy on Infectious Diseases: New Presidential Policy Calls for Coordinated Approach to Global Issue." Washington, DC: Executive Office of the President, June 12, 1996. www.fas.org/irp/offdocs/pdd_ntsc7.htm.

U.S. Congress. Senate. Committee on Appropriations. Subcommittee on Labor, Health and Human Services, Education and Related Agencies. "Prepared Testimony of Stephen Blount, Director for Global Health, CDC, May 2, 2007." Washington, DC: U.S. Department of Health and Human Services, last revised September 2010. www.dhhs.gov/asl/testify/2007/05/t20070502a.html.

U.S. Department of Defense (DOD). Global Emerging Infections Surveillance and Response System. "Fiscal Year 2008 Annual Report." Washington, DC: Government Printing Office. http://afhsc.mil/viewDocument?file=GEIS/GEISAnnRpt08.pdf.

U.S. Department of Health and Human Services. Centers for Disease Control and Prevention (CDC). "Division of Global Public Health Capacity Development 2008 Annual Report." Atlanta, GA: Centers for Disease Control and Prevention, 2009. www.cdc.gov/globalhealth/FETP/pdf/2008_annual_report_508.pdf.

———. "Global Disease Detection Policy Paper." Atlanta, GA: Centers for Disease Control and Prevention, June 2008. www.cdc.gov/cogh/pdf/GDD_at_a_Glance_2008.pdf.

———. "Global Disease Detection Program: Monitoring and Evaluation Report 2006–2008." Atlanta, GA: Centers for Disease Control and Prevention, June 2009. www.cdc.gov/globalhealth/GDD/pdf/GDD_m&e.pdf.

———. "Global Disease Detection Program, Fact Sheet: GDD Accomplishments." Atlanta, GA: Centers for Disease Control and Prevention, 2009. www.cdc.gov/globalhealth/GDD/pdf/accomplishments_2006-Q1and2-2009.pdf.

U.S. Department of State (Department of State). "Implementation of the Global Health Initiative: Consultation Document." February 2010. www.pepfar.gov/documents/organization/136504.pdf.

———. "The U.S. President's Emergency Plan for AIDS Relief: Five-Year Strategy." December 2009. www.pepfar.gov/strategy/document/index.htm.

U.S. General Accounting Office (GAO). "Challenges in Improving Infectious Disease Surveillance Systems." GAO-01-722. Washington, DC: Government Printing Office, August 2001. www.gao.gov/new.items/d01722.pdf.

U.S. Government Accountability Office (GAO). "Global Health: U.S. Agencies Support Programs to Build Overseas Capacity for Infectious Disease Surveillance." Statement of David Gootnik, director, International Affairs and Trade. GAO-08-138T. Washington, DC: Government Printing Office, October 4, 2007. www.gao.gov/new.items/d08138t.pdf.

United Nations Development Program. *Human Development Report 1994.* New York: Oxford University Press, 1995.

Upton, Maureen T. "Global Public Health Trumps the Nation-State." *World Policy Journal* 21, no. 3 (Fall 2004): 73–78.

Walt, Gill, and Kent Buse. "Global Cooperation in International Public Health." In *International Public Health: Diseases, Programs, Systems, and Policies*, edited by Michael H. Merson, Robert E. Black, and Anne J. Mills, 649–80. Sudbury, MA: Jones and Bartlett, 2006.

Waltz, Kenneth. *Theory of International Politics.* Reading, MA: Addison-Wesley, 1979.

Wendt, Alexander. "Anarchy Is What States Make of It: The Social Construction of Power Politics." *International Organization* 46, no. 2 (Spring 1992): 391–425.

Whitman, Jim. "Global Governance as the Friendly Face of Unaccountable Power." *Security Dialogue* 33, no.1 (2002): 45–57.

World Health Organization (WHO). *World Health Report 2007*. Geneva: World Health Organization, 2007.

———. "Global Burden of Disease 2004 Update." Geneva: World Health Organization, 2008. http://whqlibdoc.who.int/publications/2008/9789241563710_eng.pdf.

Yach, Derek, and Douglas Bettcher. "The Globalization of Public Health, I: Threats and Opportunities." *American Journal of Public Health* 88, no.5 (1998): 735–44.

Yin, Robert K. *Case Study Research: Design and Methods*. Beverly Hills, CA: Sage Publications, 1989.

Zacher, Mark W. "The Transformation in Global Health Collaboration since the 1990s." in *Governing Global Health: Challenge, Response, Innovation*, edited by Andrew Fenton Cooper, John J. Kirton, and Ted Schrecker, 15–27. Burlington, VT: Ashgate Publishing, 2007.

Zacher, Mark W., and Tania J. Keefe. *The Politics of Global Health Governance: United by Contagion*. New York: Palgrave Macmillan, 2008.

Zartman, I. William. "Dialog of the Deaf, Mutual Enlightenment or Doing One's Own Thing?" Paper presented at the Annual Conference of the International Studies Association, New Orleans, LA, February 18, 2010.

INDEX

Page numbers followed by *f* and *n* indicate figures and footnotes, respectively.

About the Author

William J. Long is professor and chair at the Sam Nunn School of International Affairs at the Georgia Institute of Technology. He is the author of three books and numerous articles on conflict resolution, international cooperation, and trade and technology transfer policy. He was a Jennings Randolph fellow at the U.S. Institute of Peace in 2009–10.

USIP JENNINGS RANDOLPH FELLOWSHIP PROGRAM

This book is a fine example of the work produced by senior fellows in the Jennings Randolph fellowship program of the United States Institute of Peace. As part of the statute establishing the Institute, Congress envisioned a program that would appoint "scholars and leaders of peace from the United States and abroad to pursue scholarly inquiry and other appropriate forms of communication on international peace and conflict resolution." The program was named after Senator Jennings-Randolph of West Virginia, whose efforts over four decades helped establish the Institute.

Since 1987, the Jennings Randolph Program has played a key role in the Institute's effort to build a national center of research, dialogue, and education on critical problems of conflict and peace. Fellows come from a wide variety of academic and other professional backgrounds. They conduct research at the Institute and participate in USIP's outreach activities to policymakers, the academic community, and the American public.

The Institute awards between eight and twelve senior fellowships each year. Fellowship recipients are selected after a rigorous, multistage review that includes consideration by independent experts and professional staff at the Institute. The final authority for decisions regarding Senior Fellowship awards rests with USIP's board of directors. The Jennings Randolph Program also awards Peace Scholar dissertation fellowships to students at U.S. universities who are researching and writing doctoral dissertations on conflict and international peace and security issues.

For further information, contact the JR program at (202) 457-1700 or visit our website at www.usip.org.

United States Institute of Peace Press

Since its inception, the United States Institute of Peace Press has published over 150 books on the prevention, management, and peaceful resolution of international conflicts—among them such venerable titles as Raymond Cohen's *Negotiating Across Cultures;* John Paul Lederach's *Building Peace; Leashing the Dogs of War* by Chester A. Crocker, Fen Osler Hampson, and Pamela Aall; and *American Negotiating Behavior* by Richard H. Solomon and Nigel Quinney. All our books arise from research and fieldwork sponsored by the Institute's many programs. In keeping with the best traditions of scholarly publishing, each volume undergoes both thorough internal review and blind peer review by external subject experts to ensure that the research, scholarship, and conclusions are balanced, relevant, and sound. With the Institute's move to its new headquarters on the National Mall in Washington, D.C., the Press is committed to extending the reach of the Institute's work by continuing to publish significant and sustainable works for practitioners, scholars, diplomats, and students.

Valerie Norville
Director

About the United States Institute of Peace

The United States Institute of Peace is an independent, nonpartisan institution established and funded by Congress. The Institute provides analysis, training, and tools to help prevent, manage, and end violent international conflicts, promote stability, and professionalize the field of peacebuilding.

Chairman of the Board: J. Robinson West
Vice Chairman: George E. Moose
President: Richard H. Solomon
Executive Vice President: Tara Sonenshine
Chief Financial Officer: Michael Graham

Board of Directors

J. Robinson West (Chair), Chairman, PFC Energy
George E. Moose (Vice Chairman), Adjunct Professor of Practice, The George Washington University
Anne H. Cahn, Former Scholar in Residence, American University
Chester A. Crocker, James R. Schlesinger Professor of Strategic Studies, School of Foreign Service, Georgetown University
Kerry Kennedy, President, Robert F. Kennedy Center for Justice and Human Rights
Ikram U. Khan, President, Quality Care Consultants, LLC
Stephen D. Krasner, Graham H. Stuart Professor of International Relations, Stanford University
Jeremy A. Rabkin, Professor, George Mason School of Law
Judy Van Rest, Executive Vice President, International Republican Institute
Nancy Zirkin, Executive Vice President, Leadership Conference on Civil Rights

Members ex officio

Michael H. Posner, Assistant Secretary of State for Democracy, Human Rights, and Labor

James N. Miller, Principal Deputy Under Secretary of Defense for Policy

Ann E. Rondeau, Vice Admiral, U.S. Navy; President, National Defense University

Richard H. Solomon, President, United States Institute of Peace (nonvoting)